*To all my wonderful patients who helped me create this plan
and all the readers who can now benefit from our work.*

Healing Arthritis

Your 3-Step Guide to Conquering Arthritis Naturally

Susan Blum, M.D., M.P.H.

With Michele Bender

First published in the US in 2017 by Scribner
an imprint of Simon & Schuster, Inc.
1230 Avenue of the Americas
New York, NY 10020

This edition published in Great Britain in 2017 by Orion Spring
an imprint of The Orion Publishing Group Ltd
Carmelite House, 50 Victoria Embankment
London EC4Y 0DZ

An Hachette UK Company

1 3 5 7 9 10 8 6 4 2

A CIP catalogue record for this book is
available from the British Library.

978 1 409 17945 0

Printed in Great Britain by Clays Ltd, St Ives plc

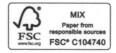

MIX
Paper from
responsible sources
FSC
www.fsc.org   FSC® C104740

ORION
SPRING

www.orionbooks.co.uk

Contents

Foreword
Why Is Gut Health So Important?

One of the most prominent focuses of health in the twenty-first century is gut health. Having too many bad critters—bacteria and other microorganisms—hanging out in the gut has been linked to numerous medical issues, including autism, obesity, diabetes, allergies, arthritis, autoimmune disorders, depression, and certain types of cancer, heart disease, fibromyalgia, eczema, and asthma. New links between chronic illness and an imbalanced microbiome (also known as gut bacteria) emerge almost every day, and the connection between the gut and inflammatory arthritis of all types is no exception.

While Western medicine has greatly advanced in treating acute disease, conditions that are easily fixed with a pill like an antibiotic, we've failed miserably in addressing chronic illness, health issues that linger because they have lifestyle issues like diet and stress as the root cause. In the mid-nineteenth century, the French microbiologist and chemist Louis Pasteur, best known for developing the process of pasteurization, discovered the bug, or microbe, that causes infections; about seventy-five years later, a Scottish biologist named Alexander Fleming developed antibiotics to cure them. This simple cause-effect "cure"—single bug, single disease, and single drug—might work for infection, but not so much for chronic disease.

Ever since, we have been searching for cures for chronic diseases (including cardiovascular and autoimmune disease and dementia), yet we can't find them! Medicine's history has become the pursuit of a holy grail: a pill for every ill. *This failed approach will continue to fail because chronic disease results from the complex interaction of our genes, lifestyle, and environment.* There is no miracle cure. Instead, we need a well-rounded, permanent lifestyle approach.

Many scientists have started referring to the gut as our "second brain," an idea reflected in amazing books such as *The Good Gut* by Justin and Erica Sonnenburg, Ph.D., *Brain Maker* by David Perlmutter, M.D., *The Microbiome Solution* by Robynne Chutkan, M.D., and *The Gut Balance Revolution* by Gerard E. Mullin, M.D. Having a healthy gut should mean more to you than being annoyed by a little bloating or heartburn. It becomes central to your entire health and connected to everything that happens in your body. That's why, like Dr. Blum and, similar to the program she lays out in *Healing Arthritis*, I almost always start treating my patients' chronic health problems by fixing their guts first.

You can begin to understand the importance of gut health when you consider that your gut contains many trillions of bacteria—*three pounds'* worth—made up of one thousand different species. Your body has about twenty thousand genes but two million (or more) bacterial genes!

Altogether, your gut is a huge chemical factory that helps to digest food, manufacture vitamins, regulate hormones, excrete toxins, and produce healing compounds, among other functions. Intestinal health could be defined as the optimal digestion, absorption, and assimilation of food. But that is a big job that depends on many other factors. For example, the bugs in your gut are like a rain forest: a diverse and interdependent ecosystem. They must be in balance for you to be healthy. Too many of the wrong ones (such as parasites, yeasts, or "bad" bacteria) or *not enough* of the good ones (*Lactobacillus* or *Bifidobacteria*) can seriously damage your health.

Dr. Susan Blum's groundbreaking book *Healing Arthritis* is a powerful guide to self-healing, showing how you can address the root causes of disease, reduce inflammation, and heal your joint pain. She lays out a clear road map to recovery for the millions of people suffering needlessly from arthritis and provides solutions for healing the gut and changes in diet, supplements, and life balance that can help people manage and even reverse these conditions. Dr. Blum's desire to find these answers was fueled by her own struggle with arthritis, a condition that she has treated successfully and recovered from by using the program described in this book.

Remember, optimal gut balance begins with a diet rich in fiber, healthy protein, and healthy fats. Good fats, including omega-3 fats and monounsaturated fats—from sources such as extra-virgin olive oil, avocados, and almonds—improve healthy gut flora, while inflammatory fats like omega-6 vegetable oils promote the growth of bad bugs that cause weight gain and disease. Lack of sleep also contributes to gut imbalance, so be sure to get seven to eight hours of quality sleep. Additionally, your gut flora listen to and are influenced by your thoughts and feelings, so it's important to practice your favorite stress reduction activities daily. You will find an easy-to-follow diet guide and ideas for relaxation practices in the pages that follow. If you suffer from any type of arthritis or inflammation and are looking for a treatment approach that offers an option to medication by addressing the root causes, this book is for you.

Mark Hyman, M.D., medical director at
Cleveland Clinic's Center for Functional Medicine,
founder of the UltraWellness Center, and a ten-time
number one *New York Times* bestselling author

Introduction

Here's a sobering statistic: approximately one in four people have arthritis at this very moment! That's more than 54 million American adults, which is more than 22 percent of the US population. And that's not all. By the year 2030, this number is estimated to skyrocket to 580 million people across the globe ages eighteen and older. (I know it's hard to believe, since arthritis is often viewed as an old person's disease.) Two-thirds of these sufferers will be women. People with arthritis commonly experience such severe joint pain and inflammation that almost half of those who've been diagnosed report physical limitations as a result. Unfortunately, this affects their ability to be physically active, which further increases their risk of other health issues like diabetes, obesity, and heart disease.

Of course, these statistics are shocking, but when you're living with arthritis, statistics don't matter. The quality of your *one, singular* life does. As a medical doctor who has been practicing functional medicine for almost two decades and is now a leading expert in this field, I have seen hundreds of people devastated by arthritis, a condition characterized by chronic pain and swelling in one or more joints. I saw this frequently when I was a solo practitioner and see it even more now as the founder and director of the Blum Center for Health in Rye Brook, New York.

Because I have treated thousands of patients with inflammatory conditions, including every kind of arthritis, I have found that functional medicine offers a better way to heal the *cause* of this potentially crippling joint disease than conventional medicine does. Functional medicine is an approach that considers the *whole* person, not just his or her symptoms. I think of functional medicine as a specialty within the field of integrative medicine, which includes every healing modality that can be added to your treatment program. These include therapies such as acupuncture, homeopathy, mind-body medicine, and craniosacral therapy. I often say that a functional medicine expert is like a medical detective gathering all the clues from your past (where you grew up, your family situation, traumatic events, your health history, and so on) and your present (your environment, social life, stress level, relationships, diet—not only what you eat but also its quality—fitness regimen, sleep habits, and symptoms, among other important factors). Armed with this information, he or she then tries to uncover how and why your body is not functioning well (hence the term *functional* medicine). You can see that it is another way of viewing disease and another approach in the clinical practice of medicine.

On the other hand, conventional medicine typically focuses on the symptoms of arthritis and relies on strong painkillers and immune-suppressing medicines to mask those symptoms. Yes, these medications may temporarily reduce your discomfort, and they are very helpful and necessary if you are experiencing a flare-up of severe pain. However, they don't target the underlying disease. One of my favorite ways to explain this is with an analogy made by Sidney Baker, M.D., a well-known preventive medicine specialist who is often called the father of functional medicine. He said, "If you are sitting on a tack, the answer is not to treat the pain. The solution is to find the tack and remove it."

So when it comes to arthritis, the goal is find the "tack" (or tacks) that are causing your painful, often debilitating symptoms and pull them out. In this book, I will show you where they are and how to remove them.

Another serious downside to medications is that they damage the gut. Your gut is your entire gastrointestinal tract: from your mouth, to your stomach, and ending in your small and large intestines. Amazingly, it has the surface area of a tennis court. Since 70 percent of your immune system lives in your gut, impairing it can have a serious negative impact on your health, such as making your arthritis worse and triggering inflammation and autoimmune diseases, among other conditions. Your gut is a good example of an important tack that must be treated in order for your arthritis to get better.

With the 2013 launch of my first book, *The Immune System Recovery Plan*, I made many appearances on *The Dr. Oz Show* and other media outlets to share my approach to treating inflammatory diseases. As a result, my medical practice had an astounding increase in patients with these conditions. But even more astounding was that most of these people had arthritis! A large number of them had rheumatoid arthritis (RA), many had psoriatic arthritis (PsA), and others were battling various autoimmune diseases, such as lupus (the full name of which is systemic lupus erythematosus) and Sjögren's syndrome, which cause arthritis *symptoms*. Then there were patients who had joint pain and swelling but hadn't been diagnosed definitively with any of these conditions, in addition to many with osteoarthritis (OA), whose pain was triggered by underlying inflammation.

As I worked closely with these patients to help them get well again and improve the quality of their lives, it became clear that those with arthritis needed their own unique program—one that specifically addressed joints and, based on the latest research, focused on treating the gut. I also realized that people with chronic inflammatory conditions needed a program that offered *permanent healing and good health, and helped them finish what they started*. Since my first book, an array of new research has confirmed what we in functional medicine have been doing with our patients for years: focusing on the gut as the origin of arthritis and inflammation. Also in that time, I've learned so much valuable information about preventing the disease from relapsing. While I still view *The Immune System Recovery Plan* as the gold standard in treating all autoimmune and inflammatory conditions, I created an innovative and *specific* arthritis program that I will share in *Healing Arthritis*. I know this program works because I've used it with all of these patients in my practice. I also know it works because I used it to cure my *own* arthritis.

In my last book, I shared the story of how I healed myself from Hashimoto's thyroiditis. While curing this autoimmune condition of the thyroid gland, the functional medicine approach that I followed also resolved issues such as high mercury levels in my blood and the bloating and constipation that had plagued me since childhood. That therapeutic journey played a crucial role in creating the approach that I detailed in *The Immune System Recovery Plan.* For five years, I maintained a strong state of health using diet, exercise, and stress management techniques. My life felt balanced. *I* felt balanced. But as John Lennon sang in "Beautiful Boy," "Life is what happens to you while you're busy making other plans." Well, this is where my life intervened with not one but two major, devastating events.

First, my nineteen-year-old son had a serious skateboarding accident that caused a terrible traumatic brain injury. Spending nights by his hospital bedside, filled with panic, was one of the worst experiences of my life. Then there were the weeks, months, and years of angst as he struggled to regain all of his functionality. When this happened, I had just opened the Blum Center for Health, where, under one roof, my patients could receive cutting-edge functional medicine treatment while also learning how to make the lifestyle changes necessary for their recovery. To do this, we offer everything from a cooking school to a mind-body-spirit center. As if I didn't have enough on my plate, I also was writing my first book. Though opening the Blum Center for Health and becoming an author were thrilling experiences, both were huge undertakings, and even good stress is, well, stress.

I was so busy that I stopped meditating regularly, something that had benefited me for years. Then I fell off my clean diet wagon by eating small amounts of dairy and gluten and drinking more alcohol and coffee. To make matters worse, my calming and consistent regimen of exercise, yoga, and long nature walks became less and less frequent. I had stopped taking care of myself.

Now, if my son's accident had been the only major life event, I'm confident that I would have eventually come back to my healthy senses and returned to the excellent self-care I'd been practicing for years. But then my father died suddenly of a massive stroke. The shock of both his passing away so unexpectedly at the age of seventy-seven and the conflict among my mother and siblings that occurred after he was gone was extremely painful. What followed was a very intense year. Like many women, I knew my family needed me, so I held it together in order to help everyone else. I kept working, seeing patients, and running the Blum Center for Health. I held my emotions in check as I cared for my children, soothed their sadness about losing the grandfather they loved so much, and worked with my mother and siblings to deal with all the issues that arise after a loved one dies.

But once the acute traumas had passed and my family seemed okay, the after-effects of stress began to appear as symptoms revealing that my physical body had been jolted. My constipation and bloating were back, and I noticed that, off and on, three of my fingers hurt when I bent or pressed them and occasionally appeared swollen. I didn't pay much attention, though. That was until I woke up one morning, and my left eye was bright red and painful. *This* really jolted me. After a trip to the eye doctor, I learned that I had episcleritis, an inflammatory disease that affects the episclera, a thin layer of tissue that forms part of the white of the eye. After doing some research, I discovered this condition can be associated with inflammatory arthritis, especially rheumatoid arthritis.

I believe my episcleritis was brought on by the traumatic stress I experienced. Trauma and stress are parts of life. We lose parents and siblings; some lose children; many get divorced or get fired from their jobs. Not surprisingly, there is a link between trauma and disease.

You will learn about my entire journey to cure my arthritis in chapter 8, "Traumatic Stress: Fueling the Flame," and in chapter 9, "My Story: Putting It All Together," but the abridged version is that I needed to fix my gut and understand and address the trauma I had suffered. I needed to work on my emotional well-being—not only in the short term but in the long term, too, so that I would stay well *per-*

manently. I began focusing on my diet and taking specific nutritional supplements and paying attention to my mental health and stress management.

Just because I'm a doctor doesn't mean that my recovery was quick and easy. It wasn't. But working through it, along with my experiences with patients, helped me create what is now *Healing Arthritis*. The plan is so effective that I noticed a big improvement in my symptoms within the first two weeks. I felt healthier than I had in a long time—maybe ever—and it helped me make this state of well-being a permanent one. Today I no longer have symptom flare-ups and can enjoy my life—and the occasional glass of wine—and avoid a relapse of my condition. I want you to do the same.

Before I go into more detail about the Arthritis Protocol, let's talk a little bit about what arthritis is. When it comes to this condition, many people—even those who *have* it—don't actually know much about it. The biggest misconception is that it is a disease that only old people get. Unfortunately, this isn't true. From 2010 to 2012, 7.3 percent of Americans ages 18 to 44 said they were diagnosed with arthritis by their doctor. For those ages 45 to 64, this number increased to 30.3 percent, according to the US Centers for Disease Control and Prevention (CDC). This is almost one-third of middle-aged Americans! There are many kinds of arthritis, and they can be grouped into three major categories:

1. **Inflammatory Arthritis.** This category includes several autoimmune conditions, but rheumatoid arthritis is the most well known and common, affecting almost sixty-eight million people worldwide. RA is the most prevalent autoimmune disease, with an estimated 1 percent of people in the United States and the United Kingdom having it at any one time. Three times as many women suffer from this condition as men do. Within ten years of receiving a diagnosis of RA, at least 50 percent of people can't hold down a full-time job, according to the World Health Organization (WHO). This category also includes the other auto-

immune arthritis conditions psoriatic arthritis and ankylosing spondyloarthritis (AS), as well as autoimmune diseases such as lupus, Sjögren's syndrome, scleroderma, and fibromyalgia, that often have arthritis as one of the symptoms.

Then there is undifferentiated (or undiagnosed) arthritis, a growing category where none of the tests comes back positive for any specific diagnosis, and doctors can't tell you what kind of arthritis you have. As a result, undifferentiated arthritis is considered a very early stage of inflammatory arthritis. Thirty percent of people in this category will later go on to develop RA, highlighting how crucial it is to treat it with a program like mine *before* this progression occurs. (Many patients who walk into my office with undiagnosed arthritis tell me that their rheumatologists believe they have early RA and have prescribed strong medication for rheumatoid arthritis even though they haven't been diagnosed.)

2. **Osteoarthritis.** This very common type of arthritis, also referred to as degenerative joint disease (DJD), is often triggered by damage to a joint from either one major injury or repetitive use over time. These insults can be from sports (for example, years of running or playing tennis), occupational overuse (typing or desk work), or an accident (breaking your wrist in a skiing mishap). However, while injury is definitely a risk factor for OA, recent research shows that obesity, diabetes, and a diet high in sugar and inflammatory fats (saturated animal fat and processed hydrogenated oils) have an even greater impact on developing this condition as well as on your pain level. People with osteoarthritis typically have specific changes in the joints that can be seen on an X-ray.

3. **Arthritis from an Infection.** This can be bacterial (Lyme disease, for instance), viral, or a reaction to an infection somewhere else in the body (reactive arthritis). In this type of arthritis, we treat the underlying infection. This is not the form of arthritis that I am discussing in this book, but I will mention it

briefly when we talk about how to know which kind of arthritis you have.

My Arthritis Protocol focuses on inflammatory arthritis and OA and tells you how to make sure you don't have arthritis from an infection. In my experience with patients, these different kinds of arthritis can sometimes happen together in the same joint, and I have seen OA turn into RA because forces within the body trigger additional inflammation. The bottom line: inflammation in the body exacerbates joint symptoms. Therefore, no matter what kind of arthritis you have, my program will help you feel better and reduce your need for medication.

How Does *Healing Arthritis* Work?

Over many years of treating and following my patients, and in dealing with my own autoimmune disease, I've realized that people usually can do what's needed short term. The problem is that after the initial kick start, and once they begin to feel better, they need a program that will help them be more resilient—so that when life events come along, they don't become sick again. *Healing Arthritis* will show you what it takes to break the vicious cycle of inflammation and get off the stress-gut-arthritis merry-go-round permanently by taking you on your own journey of self-discovery, self-care, and healing. Also, woven throughout the book are stories of real people and how I worked with them to treat their different types of arthritis, including my own. I will explain their histories, struggles, successes, and specific supplement programs in detail. My goal is to help you recognize yourself among the various patients' stories and give you inspiration and hope that, yes, you *can* get better.

Part 1, "What Kind of Arthritis Do You Have?," reviews the different types of arthritis: what they are, what research suggests causes each one, and what we know about treatment options. I review all types of arthritis because I believe it is critical for you to know *why* you have arthritis. Furthermore, even though your doctor might not know all of the latest research, we *do* know *a lot* about the causes of inflammation and joint pain. The goal of this book is to offer a treatment plan that fixes the underlying causes of your arthritis, which is the only way to be cured permanently. As a result, it is important that you learn the scientific evidence behind the program in this book—or at least be aware that there *is* science behind it. I also review the different kinds of arthritis, because I want you to know what kind you have. For example, it's important to know whether you have inflammatory arthritis or osteoarthritis because, while the causes and treatments have many similarities, there are also crucial differences.

Here is how I suggest you use part 1: if you know your diagnosis, you can go straight to that chapter and skip the rest. In your chapter, you will find information about the cause of your arthritis and what tests and symptoms you can follow to check your progress. After all, helping you live a symptom-free life is the first goal. Yet, especially for people with rheumatoid arthritis, for example, the goal is also to have normal blood tests. If you know what kind of arthritis you have, then you know where to look for this information and to read the stories of people with those diagnoses, too.

In my medical practice, I see many people who don't know what kind of arthritis they have and are very confused about the different types. If you don't know your own diagnosis, then you can't know your prognosis—that is, your prospect of returning to a healthy, active life. Those of you who have arthritis but don't know what kind should read all the chapters so that you can figure this out with my help and feel less confused. Still, no matter what kind of arthritis you have, following the Arthritis Protocol will help you feel better!

Part 2, "Heal the Gut, Heal the Joints," teaches you about the connection between gut health and all types of arthritis. I will show you the proof that the root cause of your arthritis is probably in your digestive system and that healing your gut is the first step to healing your joints. Here we will also focus on *real gut treatment programs prescribed for real patients.* I will share the exact Two-Month Intensive Gut Repair treatment plans for six patients as well as for myself, with supplement details and timelines, so that you can easily follow this program for yourself. Their stories are so inspiring!

Part 3, "Treating Your Terrain," explores the role of diet, stress, and trauma on the health of your gut microbiome. The term "microbiome" refers to all the collective good bacteria—also known as flora and "healthy" bacteria—in your body. Going forward, I will refer to the microbiome as "gut bacteria." These three factors also influence the degree of inflammation in your body and your joints. I offer you a simple yet thorough review of all the research on the different types of diets and then give you a summary of the best lifelong approach to eating that is anti-inflammatory and good for your joints. Food influences your "terrain," or what I think of as the body's deepest soil, in which all of your cells either thrive or wither. Stress, too, influences this terrain. You will learn about these relationships and how stress and trauma had a big impact on the recovery progress for my patients. I will also share the stress reduction techniques that my patients used, and what you can do about eating and living in such a way to make your cells thrive.

Finally, we put it all together in part 4, "The Blum Center 3-Step Arthritis Protocol." Here you will find a guide to the definitive 3-Step Arthritis Protocol. We begin with step 1, the Two-Week Jump-Start Leaky Gut Diet for Arthritis, where you will focus solely on changing what you eat and starting a basic anti-inflammatory supplement program. Because adopting a new way of eating can be a challenge for many people, we will keep this simple and introduce new tasks with each step of the program. This will make it easy to do.

For step 2, the Two-Month Intensive Gut Repair, you will continue with the Leaky Gut Diet for Arthritis and also begin a supplement program to treat your gut. During these two months, you should notice a dramatic improvement in symptoms. While many studies show that arthritis symptoms can improve by taking probiotics, my approach to gut repair is much more comprehensive and effective than solely using these supplements, which contain live microorganisms to stimulate or maintain beneficial bacteria in the digestive tract.

Since 2013, I have been offering steps 1 and 2 on my website Blum Health MD (www.blumhealthmd.com) as a companion to my first book. (There is a similar program for the Arthritis Protocol at www.blumhealthmd.com/arthritis.) Here my staff and I have been able to work online with more than 2,500 people suffering from various autoimmune diseases. Most of the email questions we get are from people who have inflammation, especially arthritis, and who have finished these first two steps. They feel better but are not yet completely healed. Their top question is "What comes next?" The answer is step 3, the Finish-What-You-Started Six-Month Program.

Because the gut is very sensitive to the anxiety and worries of everyday life and emotional trauma, arthritis patients are extremely susceptible to relapse from stressful experiences, past or present. I've observed this so often in the many patients I've followed for several years. What most people don't realize is that stressful experiences take a toll on the body not just mentally but also physically—especially damaging the gut by knocking healthy flora levels out of balance. One distinctive element of the Finish-What-You-Started Six-Month Program is learning to address these issues in a comprehensive way. This is crucial for permanent gut and joint repair and to help prevent the illness from recurring, so that you can live symptom free in the long term.

Even though understanding the role of stress and trauma in your illness and learning what to do about it are essential parts of your program, I wait to introduce the mind-body program until step 3 so that you can really focus on it and make it a permanent lifestyle change. It really is that important. The Finish-What-You-Started Six-Month Program is also a time when you can begin to think about tapering off some of your medicine, which I will explain in detail later in the book.

• • •

As I mentioned, since *The Immune System Recovery Plan* was published, there has been an explosion in research on the connection between gut health and joint health, and this was just the beginning. There have also been new, reliable studies on the healthy bacteria that live in and on your body. On the skin, in the lungs, and in the gut, these bacteria protect us from the environment, and studies continue to prove that they influence every aspect of our health. The gut bacteria, which are estimated to number up to a hundred trillion—about the same as the number of cells in your entire body—live inside the gastrointestinal tract and play a key role in strengthening your immune system. Almost daily, a new study or story confirms what we in the functional medicine world already know about the importance of the gut bacteria: imbalances in this bacteria are a direct driver of arthritis—and, conversely, you can cure arthritis by repairing the gut bacteria. An imbalance can be an overgrowth of bad bacteria or not enough of the good bacteria. What is essential to realize is that the inflammation may start in the gut but then shows up in other places, such as joints, muscles, the brain, and fat cells.

With a growing epidemic of gut problems in our country, it's not surprising that inflammatory arthritis is also on the rise, as the two go hand in hand. It is crucial that we pay close attention to this gut-arthritis connection and repair the gut to effectively treat arthritis. Just about every new patient walking into my office has constipation, gas, bloating, gastroesophageal reflux disease (GERD, also known as acid reflux, a condition where your stomach contents move into your throat, causing a burning sensation), heartburn, or a diagnosis of irritable bowel syndrome (IBS). Plus, in the past few years, several new conditions have emerged, such as a recently discovered kind of IBS called small intestinal bacterial overgrowth (SIBO), a chronic disorder of the small intestine. Many experts believe that SIBO is now more common because of our society's rampant use of antacids and proton pump inhibitors—medicines that lower stomach acid to treat symptoms of heartburn and reflux but have adverse side effects.

Much of this new research and insight has caught the attention of both the mainstream medical community and the media. I believe that it won't be long until we make the connection between the gut and *every* part of the body, but, at this point, I'm content that the link between the gut and inflammatory arthritis is very strong and more widely disseminated.

In the Arthritis Protocol, I will highlight and explain this new research and its relevance in a way that is simple and easy to understand. These advancements in the few years since my first book have opened the door for, and led the way to, improved functional medicine treatments and outcomes. The Arthritis Protocol combines my analysis of the newest research and treatments with my extensive experience on repairing the gut. My patients' improved health and great results are clear evidence that the Arthritis Protocol works and works well.

All my arthritis patients begin on a treatment plan like the one in the Arthritis Protocol. However, after the first three months, each person sets his or her own course for what comes next. This is where patients need help navigating how to continue with the gut treatment and learning how to prevent their unpredictable lives from causing imbalance, symptoms, and disease *again*. The reality is, we don't live in a vacuum. We live go-go-go lives, don't get enough sleep, experience distressing events, and go on vacation and celebrate birthdays, among many other things. The Arthritis Protocol will be your detailed road map through this uncharted territory. To guide you, I'll share the stories of eleven real patients who have arthritis. Since life affects the gut so powerfully and the gut affects inflammation so intimately, understanding this balance is critical in order to build resiliency. This information is best illustrated through the eyes of people actually suffering from arthritis, as each has had a unique but overlapping set of circumstances and triggers for the vicious stress-gut-arthritis cycle. Also, each patient has followed a slightly different path to getting better. The goal in sharing a variety of stories is that you will find elements that resonate with you and help you on your personal journey. Additionally, my hope is that you will find inspiration in seeing how real people have progressed through the Arthritis Protocol and emerged stronger and healthier than before. The bottom line? You *can* have permanent improvement in your arthritis, and you *should* have hope that you can improve the quality of your life. Let's get started!

PART 1

What Kind of Arthritis Do You Have?

There are more than a dozen different kinds of arthritis, and to understand your best treatment, it's important to know which kind you have. In my medical practice, I generally see three main categories of arthritis, and each is approached differently. The first, inflammatory arthritis, includes RA and the spondyloarthritides (psoriatic arthritis and ankylosing spondyloarthritis), as well as arthritis associated with other autoimmune diseases, such as Sjögren's syndrome and lupus. An autoimmune disease is when your immune cells attack the tissues of your own body, damaging them and causing inflammation. There are more than a hundred different autoimmune diseases, which were the focus on my first book, The Immune System Recovery Plan.

Second, there is osteoarthritis, the most common form of arthritis and a leading cause of disability in the United States and around the world. Finally, there is a very large category that includes all types of infections that can trigger arthritis; for example, Lyme disease, and viruses such as parvovirus and hepatitis B. While this book will not focus on treating arthritis from infections, they can complicate or interfere with the physician's ability to make a definitive diagnosis, so it is very important to know about them so that you can seek help from your doctor to have the infection treated.

In the conventional medical world, the approach to inflammatory arthritis is to determine first if you have rheumatoid arthritis because it is the most aggressive and potentially damaging inflammatory arthri-

tis. For that reason, the goal is to make the diagnosis and catch RA early so that you can begin treatment ASAP. This is also why anyone with inflamed joints in the hands, wrists, feet, or toes should be checked for this disease. Therefore, I will begin with RA and then review the other possibilities.

CHAPTER I

Rheumatoid Arthritis

When I first met June, she was a sixty-eight-year-old who had been diagnosed with RA two years earlier. She was also at the absolute end of her rope. Even though her doctor had put her on three strong, commonly prescribed RA medicines—prednisone, methotrexate, and most recently hydroxychloroquine (also known as Plaquenil)—and she was taking over-the-counter Aleve daily, the pain in her hands was so severe that this working, married mother of four couldn't open a water bottle, carry a book, or brush her hair. Something as simple as putting on a bra was so excruciating that she needed her husband's help getting dressed each morning. For an independent, busy woman, this was devastating. Her other symptoms, such as fatigue and knee pain, also hadn't resolved with conventional treatment.

Unfortunately, June's story isn't unique, and it is what leads frustrated RA sufferers to seek out experts like me in a last-ditch effort to find hope. Using the functional medicine approach, I have helped thousands of people with inflammatory conditions reduce their pain and get back to fully living lives that have been marginalized because of their symptoms. This is what happened with June.

Within three months of our first visit, she was able to open water bottles more easily, brush her hair, and get dressed on her own with minimal pain. Her knee issues improved, and her energy level was higher than it had been in months—maybe even years. She was also able to reduce her prednisone dose by half and was taking Aleve only three or four days per week instead of every day. But this was just the beginning. June's health continued to improve as she followed the Arthritis Protocol, which I'll explain later in the book. I share June's story because it shows that with patience and perseverance, there *is* hope for everyone with this condition. There *is* hope that you can be symptom free, and there *is* hope that you can live a full life rather than sit on the sidelines.

I think of RA as the Queen of Arthritis. Like the queen in chess, rheumatoid arthritis has the ability to inflict the most damage. And like the queen in chess, who is the only one who can move in all directions, RA has an unpredictable ability to cause a wide range of symptoms. The condition is characterized by chronic joint inflammation with severe pain and swelling, joint damage, and disability. It can also come with muscle pain and soreness, which clearly reflects that this is a systemwide disease that produces inflammation throughout the body. Typically, RA affects multiple joints in the hands, feet, and wrists, a condition called polyarthritis. If left unchecked, cartilage and bone can erode, causing joint destruction, and tendons and ligaments can stretch, causing deformity. In the worst case, you can lose total function of the joint. This quick progression and severity of symptoms creates a lot of fear and panic in both doctors and their patients, which is why strong medications are often prescribed very quickly.

Fatigue is another huge issue for many RA sufferers. Often you wake up feeling exhausted even though you've gotten a good night's sleep, and you can't get through your day-to-day activities. For example, you can't concentrate at work, take the yoga class you used to love, or find the energy to play with your children. Over time, missing out on these simple but essential parts of life can leave you feeling depressed. Also over time, you forget what it feels like to *not* be fatigued. For example, after six months of working with me, June remarked that her energy level was so much higher and that she hadn't even realized how fatigued she had been for years until now. After reviewing many studies on RA and fatigue, researchers at the University of Twente in the Netherlands found that pain was the symptom associated most often with intense fatigue. Not surprisingly, losing some physical functioning and any kind of disability were also linked to fatigue, as was depression. Results on sleep were mixed, with some studies showing a connection, while other studies did not. This surprised me because I often find that people who have painful arthritis sleep poorly, which leaves them feeling exhausted. Interestingly, RA sufferers who felt they had inadequate support from friends and family or more social stress also reported higher levels of fatigue.[1] (The best way to treat inflammation may be a topic of debate, but supporting loved ones when they're not feeling well is something that we can all do for one another.) Sometimes the pain, fatigue, and other symptoms are so bad that you can't function, as in June's situation, and sometimes they are mild and easier to live with. More often they are somewhere in between.

What Causes RA?

Amazingly, the cause of this disease is unknown. However, it is generally accepted that certain microbial infections in people who are genetically susceptible to RA can trigger this autoimmune disorder. One of these is a bacterium called *Proteus mirabilis*, which, if it infects the GI tract or the urinary tract, is believed to trigger RA. Researchers at Griffith University in Queensland, Australia, concluded that the best way to prevent and treat RA would be to limit the levels of this type of bacteria in the gastrointestinal tract and to treat urinary tract infections. When *P. mirabilis* that make their home in the gut interact with the immune system and trigger the production of antibodies, it can begin a cascade of autoimmune events associated with RA. I think of antibodies as guided missiles that your immune cells release to attack a foe that triggers an alarm response in your body. Research has found that using herbs as plant-based medicine to destroy these bacteria in the gut greatly reduced the production of anti-*Proteus* antibodies.[2] These same patients also had an improvement in their arthritis symptoms. This study showed clearly that treating the gut bacteria is a valid strategy for treating inflammatory arthritis, and helps lay the scientific foundation for my gut-repair approach in the Arthritis Protocol.

Bacteria, fungi, and viruses have also been studied as potential causes of RA. In addition to *Proteus*, bacterial pathogens such as *Coxiella burnetii*, oral anaerobic bacteria, and the species *Staphylococcus, Streptococcus, Neisseria, Haemophilus*, and *Mycoplasma* have all been reported as causes of RA, although there has not been enough strong evidence to prove this.

Researchers at Baqiyatallah University of Medical Sciences in Tehran, Iran, studied the fluid inside the joints of people with RA, looking for different species of *Mycoplasma*. Twenty-three percent had one species, 17.5 percent had another species, and 10 percent had yet another, showing that it isn't the cause of RA in everyone but it could be in some people. This also supports the idea that infections could be one of RA's triggers and that treating the infections or helping your immune system fight the infections better by repairing and strengthening the gut bacteria is a strategy worth incorporating in a comprehensive and effective approach to preventing and treating this condition.[3]

For each person, genetics explains only about 20 percent of why he or she developed rheumatoid arthritis. External triggers are responsible for the other 80 percent. Other than infections, these include smoking tobacco; a diet high in foods that induce inflammation, such as sugar, fried food, red meat, dairy, and alcohol; severe, ongoing chronic stress; a sudden traumatic event (a huge stressor that happens all at once and overwhelms the body); a physical injury; and exposure to environmental toxins like mercury in fish, and other toxins like pesticides and plastics.[4] Like most chronic inflammatory conditions, it is believed to be caused by an interaction of these potential triggers in people who are genetically susceptible.

Researchers at the University of Rome in Italy are working to identify a specific genetic pattern that is associated with RA, because this would help us identify people who are more likely to develop this disease.[5] As research continues to unfold, identifying more genes has the potential to help create specific treatments targeted to these genes. Until then, we have to target the external triggers. Keep in mind that even though we might not know all the specific genes at play, they are still influencing your arthritis. You may experience the stress of a divorce and never develop RA, while this same traumatic event will trigger the disease in your best friend because she is genetically sensitive to developing it. Or a divorce could bring on a mild case of arthritis for you and a more severe one for your friend. This is why we need to pinpoint *your* potential triggers. Once we do that, we can fix the underlying problem and live symptom free. In *Healing Arthritis,* we will work on fixing these triggers together.

Autoimmunity and Oxidative Stress

RA is an autoimmune disease in which the cells of the immune system attack the tissue inside the joints, triggering inflammation. Researchers at the University Medical Center Utrecht in the Netherlands studied what happens in the joints to produce inflammation. If you're healthy, the soft tissue between the joint capsule and cavity—called the synovial membrane—secretes a fluid that lubricates the joint. When you have RA, this soft tissue becomes inflamed, which can cause cells in the area to overgrow and thicken, a condition called hyperplasia. Eventually this can lead to cartilage and bone destruction. This process is believed to start when different kinds of immune cells migrate and accumulate in the joints. Some of these cells make antibodies that attack the joints as part of the autoimmune process and trigger ongoing inflammation. Inflammatory chemicals called cytokines are also released, both in the joints and throughout the body. If your immune system is balanced and healthy, this response is eventually turned off by T regulator cells, which are part of your army of immune cells. In people with RA, however, it appears that these

T cells are impaired, which makes the pain, inflammation, and other symptoms worse.[6]

This immune attack also causes oxidative stress, a very normal process that results when the cells of your body do their daily work. As they go about this, they make molecules called free radicals, which I think of as sparks or minifires. Your body's antioxidant defense systems then quench these free radicals. Low levels of oxidative stress are actually useful for the body's routine activities. Because disarming free radicals is a normal process, nature gave us antioxidants in the food we eat, especially in fruits and vegetables, a variety of which are represented by their bright and varied colors. Antioxidants include vitamins like A, C, and E, as well as colorful compounds called phytonutrients, with names you might recognize, such as resveratrol in red grapes. This is why you should eat antioxidant-rich foods daily in order to give your body the fire extinguisher to put out the sparks. In contrast, if you don't consume enough antioxidants to keep up with all the sparks, eventually the free radicals win, the sparks become a fire, and this fuels inflammation, tissue damage, and, ultimately, disease. *In particular, oxidative stress can affect your immune cells because they are very active and produce and release free radicals when doing their daily work protecting you.* This is how we believe RA and other inflammatory arthritis conditions take hold and flourish.

Many, many studies have shown that people with RA have increased levels of molecules called reactive oxygen species (ROS), a family of free radicals that have the potential to damage lipids (fats that are part of every cell and also include cholesterol, which is the way the body transports fat from one cell to another), proteins (an essential foundation of all your tissues, including the joints), and DNA (the genetic code in every cell) in joint tissue. Under normal conditions, ROS are controlled by a variety of your body's antioxidant defense systems. In people with RA, however, the antioxidants can't keep up, the free radicals run amok, and this damages tissue. When combined with the ongoing attack on your joints by your immune system, this high level of oxidative stress continues to fuel inflammation, and together this whole process can ultimately lead to the destruction of bone, joints, and articular (joint) cartilage.

Researchers from Aligarh Muslim University in India compared oxidative stress in RA sufferers with healthy individuals unaffected by this disease. They found that the people with rheumatoid arthritis exhibited high levels of oxidative stress, including increased production of free radicals, and damage to the fats (lipid peroxidation), proteins (protein oxidation), and DNA in their tissues from these free radicals. Additionally, people with RA had impaired antioxidant defense systems and low levels of two specific antioxidants: glutathione and vitamin C. Glutathione, a powerful antioxidant made by the body, is probably the most important antioxidant because it functions inside all your cells to protect you from ROS damage. Interestingly, the subjects who'd had rheumatoid arthritis the longest were found to have higher levels of oxidative stress and lower levels of antioxidants— and the higher the levels of oxidative stress, the worse their pain and disability.[7]

Research continues to support the idea that oxidative stress is a hallmark of RA. According to experts at Autonomous University of Chihuahua in Mexico, free radicals appear to directly damage joint cartilage, which shows that there is oxidative stress in the synovium of the joint itself.[8] They also found that free radicals play a role in triggering the body's inflammatory and immune responses and that people who experienced this also had low levels of antioxidants, including glutathione, vitamin E, beta-carotene, and vitamin A. It's unclear whether the low antioxidant levels are the result of the arthritis or were there before, perhaps allowing the oxidative stress to get worse, like a runaway train that can't stop. In either scenario, consuming enough antioxidants through diet, and perhaps initially through supplements, is ultimately the key to reversing the inflammation and pain of this condition.

Your antioxidant system uses many different enzymes (a protein that acts as a catalyst for chemical reactions in your body), vitamins, minerals, and amino acids (the building blocks of the protein that we eat) to manage oxidative stress, which is why your diet is so important and a lack of these nutrients may contribute to the onset of your arthritis. (Chapter 7, "Food and Fire," will teach you how to bolster your antioxidant system through your diet.) Environmental exposures and triggers can also add oxidative stress, and for some people, this is worse than others, creating bigger fires that require even more antioxidants. Eventually, if the flames grow too big, the result is runaway inflammation and tissue damage.

Environmental triggers of oxidative stress are the same as those that cause an impaired immune system: the wrong food or not enough of the right food, emotional stress and trauma, impaired gut health, and toxins and infections. All of these increase free radicals, something I talk about at length in my first book, *The Immune System Recovery Plan*. There I focus on steps to treat and remove these triggers so that the immune system begins to work properly again. Through this process, we are also treating and reducing oxidative stress. The Arthritis Protocol focuses on healing your gut, changing your diet, and helping you understand the trauma and stress in your life in order to reduce oxidative stress and inflammation and improve your health permanently.

Environmental toxins also generate high levels of free radicals, causing oxidative stress in the body. The most common ones that have been studied with respect to autoimmunity are heavy metals, pesticides, and smoking. Whether you develop symptoms or disease from these toxins is a balance between your genetic susceptibility, the magnitude of your exposure, and how well your diet and lifestyle help you keep up with your high need for antioxidants.[9] Therefore, if you have RA or any inflammatory arthritis, you have too much oxidative stress, so you need to pay attention to your toxin exposure as part of your treatment. The Leaky Gut Diet for Arthritis in chapter 10 will help you lower your toxin load in addition to reducing inflammation and pain. Because toxins are such an important trigger for autoimmunity in general, I offer an in-depth detox program in *The Immune System Recovery Plan*. Here we focus on the gut-arthritis connection because research has recently shown that this is the most important trigger of all for this condition. We will explore this further in chapter 5, "The Gut-Arthritis Connection," and chapter 6, "How to Heal the Gut."

Before we move on, just one more thing: if you have RA and smoke cigarettes, you must stop if you want to get better. There is a clear connection between tobacco use and RA that is unlike any other form of arthritis or any other toxin. Smoking is considered the number one trigger for RA because it brings many toxins into the body—such as the heavy metal cadmium—and increases oxidative stress. Plus, studies have shown that cigarette smoking may trigger one of the antibodies associated with RA.[10] Smoking not only increases your RA risk but also boosts your chances of having a more severe form of the disease and less improvement with treatment.[11]

In functional medicine, the practitioner spends a lot of time learning about your past *and* your present in order to figure out what has likely caused *your* arthritis and then create a personalized treatment plan. When I did this with June, I realized that her triggers were probably a damaged gut, toxin exposure, and stress, which can cause damage to the gut bacteria and intestinal lining. Although she had no trauma in her early years, she had some in her adult life. The oldest of June's four children has special needs, and her middle child had to have major surgery several years ago. Also, her job as a teacher was clearly stressful and affecting her RA, because her symptoms seemed to fluctuate with the school calendar. When we first started working together, it was the end of the school year, and her symptoms improved rapidly over the summer. But then September rolled around, and within a few months, she had a flare-up. The good news was that after another ten months of working together, the following fall when she returned to school, she did not suffer a flare-up.

"Two years earlier, I was hobbling to my classroom and couldn't hold a pencil," says June. "I can now walk, carry my books and papers, and move things around my classroom without pain. This feels so unusual for me that I keep waiting for the other shoe to drop." It never did.

While each person has a unique set of circumstances that triggers his or her arthritis, we know that the most important underlying foundational cause for arthritis is a problem in your gut. An imbalance in your gut bacteria can lead to a condition called leaky gut syndrome. In turn, this can trigger autoimmunity, systemwide inflammation, and oxidative stress, and is at the core of the problem for most of my patients. Part 2, "Heal the Gut, Heal the Joints," explores what we know about how problems in the gut cause problems in the joints, and our discussion about what causes RA continues there.

Diagnosing Rheumatoid Arthritis

Prior to 2010, rheumatologists followed criteria from 1987 that focused on symptoms of long-term disease such as rheumatoid nodules (bumps that can develop around an inflamed joint), joint damage, and X-ray results to diagnose RA. But in 2010 the American College of Rheumatology (ACR) redefined the disease and updated its method for diagnosing it, so that it now centers on new antibody and inflammation lab tests and signs and symptoms of inflammation such as joint pain and swelling. Plus, unlike the criteria from 1987, you don't need to have joint damage. Not only does this updated focus make it easier for physicians to diagnose RA, it identifies people who might be in the early stages of the disease—possibly up to five years before they would meet the full criteria to be diagnosed with RA, according to research from the University of Manchester in the United Kingdom.[12]

Today there seem to be more people with RA than ever before, but it's hard to know if there actually are more cases or if people are just being diagnosed earlier.[13] Either way, these new guidelines are a positive development because they allow us to treat and reverse arthritis before it becomes damaging, whether you use conventional treatment or the functional medicine approach outlined in this book. You can see the ACR 2010 classification criteria in the sidebar, and if you have been diagnosed with RA, I suggest you add up your score so that you can follow your progress as you go through the protocol. Our goal is for your score to drop under 6, which would mean your arthritis is in remission.

AMERICAN COLLEGE OF RHEUMATOLOGY CLASSIFICATION CRITERIA:

You have rheumatoid arthritis if (1) you have inflammation in at least one joint that isn't explained by another disease and (2) score 6 or higher based on the following diagnostic criteria:

	Score	Enter your score:
Joints: choose one		
One large joint (shoulder, elbow, hip, knee, ankle)	0	
Two to ten large joints	1	
One to three small joints (wrist, finger, thumb, toe). In the hands, it includes the joint at the base of the fingers, the finger joint closest to your hand (proximal), and your wrist. In the feet, it includes the joint at the base of the toes, except the big toe.	2	
Four to ten small joints	3	
More than ten small and large joints	5	
Antibody testing: choose one		
Negative results for both (1) Rheumatoid factor (RF) blood test and (2) anti-citrullinated peptide antibody (ACPA) blood test	0	

(continued on next page)

	Score	Enter your score:
Low-positive result for either RF or ACPA	2	
High-positive result for either RF or ACPA*	3	
Inflammation blood tests: choose one		
Normal results for C-reactive protein (CRP) and erythrocyte sedimentation rate (ESR) blood tests	0	
Abnormal CRP or ESR	I	
Duration of symptoms (joint pain, swelling, tenderness): choose one		
Less than six weeks	0	
Six weeks or more	I	
YOUR TOTAL SCORE		

SCORING

- If your score is equal to or greater than 6, you likely have rheumatoid arthritis.
- If your score is less than 6, you don't have RA or are in remission.
- Even if your score is less than 6, you can be diagnosed with RA based on the results of your X-ray, ultrasound, MRI, or CT scan.

* A high-positive result for either RF or ACPA is defined as greater than three times the upper limit of the normal lab value.

The antibody blood tests to diagnose RA look for antibodies called rheumatoid factor (RF) and anti-citrullinated peptide antibodies (anti-CCP, or ACPA), which often appear before symptoms such as joint pain and swelling do. They help identify people who can benefit from a functional medicine treatment plan to prevent them from developing symptoms in the future. The opposite is also true. Some people actually test *negatively* for RA, but they are given an RA diagnosis because their symptoms and other results meet the ACR

2010 definition.[14] This is called seronegative RA, and even though it's believed to be an early stage of the disease, rheumatologists often prescribe methotrexate (MTX). It belongs to a class of drugs called disease-modifying anti-rheumatic drugs (DMARDs), often used to treat RA. This confuses patients because such strong medications seem like overkill for the symptoms they are experiencing and their severity.

Sherry, a patient who came to see me when she was forty years old, had just been diagnosed with RA by a rheumatologist because she'd tested positive for rheumatoid factor and had pain and swelling in four joints in her feet. She came to me because she wanted to find an answer to her problem that addressed the root cause instead of treating only symptoms with methotrexate, as her doctor had suggested. I'm always excited when I have the opportunity to work with someone who hasn't started medication, because I *know* that treating the underlying arthritis triggers with a functional medicine approach can actually cure the disease rather than mask it by temporarily alleviating symptoms. This can prevent the need for medication altogether. This happens day after day in my practice and with the other practitioners at the Blum Center for Health. The good news is that no matter where you are on the RA spectrum—whether your disease has progressed quickly like June's, or without damage and no medication like Sherry's—the Arthritis Protocol will help you reach your goals, including becoming pain free and reducing or getting off your medication. In the end, Sherry never needed medication.

It's important to know how your doctor is making your RA diagnosis because he or she will use these criteria to decide whether or not your treatment is working and if you are in remission. With my patients, I follow the 2010 ACR guidelines and suggest you do, too, for your own information while also following the Arthritis Protocol and my recommendations in this book. It will help you gauge whether your RA is improving and when you might ask your doctor about tapering and possibly even stopping your medication. However, this isn't necessary, and you can also use how you feel as a guide.

Many people wonder why their doctors send them for X-rays or other imaging tests of their hands to figure out what kind of arthritis they have or to check to see if they are getting better or worse with treatment. X-rays, CT (computed tomography) scans, MRI (magnetic resonance imaging), and ultrasound are very useful tools for evaluating joint inflammation and damage and making a diagnosis with or without the patient's meeting other ACR 2010 criteria. A skilled radiologist can differentiate between the various kinds of arthritis simply by examining these pictures, which can be very helpful when blood tests are normal.[15] The joints in people with RA are very distinct from those in people with other forms of arthritis because there can be low bone density (known as osteopenia) in the bones on either side of the joint, loss of joint space, bone erosions, and/or soft tissue swelling. In chronic disease, this can turn into a misalignment of the joint. In the feet, RA usually affects both the toe joints and the joints in the ball of the foot. If you have arthritis in your hands and feet, it's usually on both your right and left sides (symmetrical).

Imaging tests can also pick up synovitis: inflammation in the lining of the joint capsule, which seems to happen even before you experience arthritis symptoms. When researchers at the Friedrich-Alexander University of Erlangen-Nuremberg in Germany used CT scans and MRIs to image the joints of people with RA, they found that synovitis was very common in those who tested positive for antibodies but had no arthritis symptoms. They also discovered that small areas of damage were associated with later-developing RA. The study's authors concluded that inflammation develops gradually, leading to arthritis. The pain finally flares up and is felt only when a certain inflammation threshold is crossed.[16]

This and other research suggest that RA is like an iceberg: above the surface, you see only a very small piece of the iceberg, and that doesn't reflect the magnitude of what's going on underneath— especially in the time before you experience symptoms and receive a diagnosis. This strongly highlights the need for your doctor to be very aggressive with screening tests if you have arthritis, persistent fatigue, or inflammatory markers in your blood tests. If you have the latter, you *must* be treated as if you already have RA, even if you aren't experiencing any joint pain, because you can target and treat the inflammation before you ever develop arthritis symptoms and there is any permanent damage. This is the perfect time to use a functional medicine approach to resolve the arthritis even before it begins.

Early (or Seronegative) RA

It is very common to have joint pain, stiffness, or swelling that doesn't meet any of the diagnostic criteria for RA. When this happens, many rheumatologists will tell you that you have early RA, meaning that you will likely go on to develop the disease if you don't do anything. This is called seronegative because your blood tested negative for RA antibodies. In fact, 60 percent of people with early rheumatoid arthritis have a normal ESR and CRP (markers for inflammation), while 70 percent have a normal RF test and 70 percent have normal X-rays.[17] This is called a diagnosis of exclusion: first we do the detective work to rule out other possible causes, such as a virus, Lyme disease, gout, or another autoimmune disorder. (See sidebar on pages 18–20.) If we can't find anything, as long as your arthritis symptoms are in the typical RA pattern (generally fingers or toes), then you can be given this early, or seronegative, RA diagnosis.

Early RA is a cause for concern because it means that you're heading toward a full-blown version of this disease unless you do something about it. This is exactly what happened to me. When I realized that I had arthritis in my fingers, even though all my tests were normal, the fear that I could wind up with rheumatoid arthritis propelled me to commit 1,000 percent to the Arthritis Protocol. By fixing my gut, sticking with my mind-body practices, and following the Leaky Gut Diet for Arthritis, I cured the arthritis and ensured that I would never end up with RA. I will share exactly what I did in chapter 9, "My Story: Putting It All Together."

Sometimes early inflammatory arthritis comes and goes mysteriously in episodes lasting hours to days, and symptom-free periods last days to months. The attacks can happen without any obvious triggers. This type of arthritis, called palindromic arthritis, is thought to be an early form of RA even though all tests are normal. Polymyalgia rheumatica, another kind of seronegative inflammatory arthritis, appears similar to RA because there is synovitis in the smaller joints in the hands and feet. But the joint pain is much milder and usually on only one side of the body (asymmetrical), and patients experience a lot of muscle pain, too. People with these conditions should also follow the Arthritis Protocol.

DIAGNOSING ARTHRITIS AT-A-GLANCE SUMMARY

INFLAMMATORY ARTHRITIS
Rheumatoid Arthritis (RA)

- Affects small joints, usually hands and feet, on both sides of the body.
- Tests needed for diagnosis: blood tests for rheumatoid factor (RF), anti-citrullinated peptide antibodies (ACPA), erythrocyte sedimentation rate (ESR), and C-reactive protein (CRP). ACPA is the most specific for RA.

Spondyloarthritis (SA)

- Includes psoriatic arthritis and ankylosing spondylitis.
- Your other symptoms should include: psoriasis, inflammatory bowel disease, back pain, or a family history of spondyloarthritis.
- Tests needed for diagnosis: skin examination for psoriasis and blood test for the human leukocyte antigen (HLA-B27, a genetic test).

Autoimmune Disease

- Includes systemic lupus erythematosus (SLE), Sjögren's syndrome (SS), dermatomyositis, polymyositis, and scleroderma.

- Tests needed for diagnosis include: antibody blood test for antinuclear antibody (ANA), anti-double-stranded DNA (anti-dsDNA) test, the Sjögren's tests for anti-SSA and anti-SSB antibodies. (See full list of autoimmune tests on page 59.)

Arthritis of Inflammatory Bowel Disease (IBD)

- If you have a history of abdominal pain, diarrhea or blood in your stools, a gastroenterologist can make the diagnosis of IBD.

Seronegative Inflammatory Arthritis

- Also called undifferentiated arthritis or early RA.
- You are given this diagnosis if you have normal tests for RA, and tests for other types of arthritis are normal, too.
- While you can have arthritis with pain in any of the joints in your body, it is likely to be early RA if fingers and/or toes are involved.

OSTEOARTHRITIS

- Tests needed for diagnosis: an X-ray is the best way to diagnose.

INFECTIONS
Virus or Bacteria

- Usually lasts only six to eight weeks.
- Tests needed for diagnosis: blood tests for the viruses parvovirus, hepatitis, rubella, and mumps, and for the bacteria mycoplasma.
- If you have recently traveled, ask your doctor to check for the newer mosquito-borne viruses such as chikungunya.

Reactive Arthritis

- If you've recently had a urinary tract infection or any infection in your body, you can have a reactive arthritis in your joints that usually also causes pain and swelling in the soft tissue around the joints. Tests needed for diagnosis: urine, blood, or semen culture.

Lyme Arthritis

- Lyme disease is an infection you get from a tick bite. However, it is very common to get Lyme without ever seeing a tick on your skin.
- Affects the larger joints; unusual for it to cause arthritis in the fingers and toes.
- Tests needed for diagnosis: if you have any new *arthritis-like* symptoms, ask your doctor to test you for Lyme disease.

Septic Arthritis

- An infected joint.
- Tests needed for diagnosis: your doctor can use a needle to withdraw a fluid sample from the joint and culture it to find the pathogen.

OTHER CAUSES

Gout

- Uric acid crystals in the joints.
- Tests needed for diagnosis: blood test for uric acid, X-rays, and your doctor can look for crystals in the fluid of the joint.

Fibromyalgia

- No joint inflammation or synovitis.
- Tenderness is outside of the joints and in the muscles and tendons.
- Tests needed for diagnosis: there are no blood tests; the diagnosis is based on a physical examination by your doctor.

Arthritis of Sarcoidosis

- Tests needed for diagnosis: check blood levels of angiotensin-converting enzyme (ACE) and a chest X-ray to check for sarcoid, an inflammatory disease that affects multiple organs in the body, especially the lungs.[18]

Treatment for RA

If you're reading this book, medication is probably on your mind. Maybe you're using it currently, or did so in the past, or perhaps you're considering it. Here I'll briefly review the most commonly prescribed RA medications. Clearly, this is not the focus of the book or the Arthritis Protocol, but understanding your options is crucial. It's also important to know that I am not anti-medication and do believe that it has a place. For example, if your arthritis began with unbearable pain and inflammation, or you're having a severe flare-up of your pain or chronic pain that is impairing your ability to function, prescription medication will help put out those fires in the short run. It is the right choice at those moments, and I defer to your rheumatologist to guide you on the best options. But even when medication is helpful, my goal is to simultaneously quell those deepest fires so that you need medication only for the briefest amount of time. Prescriptions are more of a Band-Aid. Yes, they can ease the inflammation so that you feel better, but they don't address the actual *cause* of your arthritis. Once things have cooled off, then the functional medicine approach takes front stage.

Prescription Medication

The first line of treatment offered by rheumatologists are conventional disease-modifying anti-rheumatic drugs (DMARDs), which act on the immune system to slow the progression of arthritis. However, corticosteroids (steroids such as prednisone) are often used briefly when you're first diagnosed to get the disease and symptoms under control quickly. After this, the goal is to move off steroids as soon as possible and onto one of the DMARDs. Sometimes corticosteroids are prescribed later during treatment to tame an acute flare-up. However, in the long term, they are very damaging. They can cause serious side effects—such as osteoporosis, sarcopenia (muscle wasting), adrenal suppression (the gland that makes your own natural steroids, such as the hormone cortisol), hair loss, weight gain, and immune suppression—so it's not ideal to stay on steroids too long.

Initially, these potent anti-inflammatories work like magic to relieve pain, but the body can become dependent on them. I've had some patients who could get off steroids easily, and I've had others like June, who made two attempts without success. When she couldn't achieve this important goal without her symptoms returning, we agreed that, given all of her emotional and physical stress at work, it was not the right time to change medication. When she became my patient, I knew that she would be retiring in a year, and so we decided to wait. Once she retired, we restarted the tapering process in earnest.

Methotrexate (MTX), the most commonly used DMARD, is the cornerstone of RA treatment and often effective on its own. Although its side effects tend to be mild, the drug's effectiveness usually wears off over time, and a second medication, called a biologic DMARD, is often added. MTX impairs your body's ability to use folate, a very important B vitamin that helps decode your genes, stabilize your mood, metabolize and excrete toxins, make energy and red blood cells, and is involved in many more biochemical processes called methylation. In this way, methotrexate impairs cell proliferation and causes cell death. While the target is your immune cells, it affects every other cell in your body, too. This is why people taking MTX are always given prescription folate at the same time. Common side effects include ulcers in your mouth, an inflamed and burning tongue, gingivitis, nausea, vomiting, diarrhea, loss of appetite, sore throat, and fatigue.

Other DMARDs are hydroxychloroquine (Plaquenil), sulfasalazine (Azulfidine), and leflunomide (Arava). Plaquenil, a drug that was traditionally used to treat malaria, is not very effective on its own and is usually added to MTX. Exactly how Plaquenil helps improve arthritis symptoms isn't clear, but it is believed to inhibit antibody reactions and suppress activity of one type of immune cell. It may also have a positive influence on gut flora. The drug, while usually well tolerated, can give rise to adverse side effects such as nausea and vomiting, headache, dizziness, irritability, muscle weakness, and potential damage to the retina of your eyes, which requires ongoing visits to your ophthalmologist, as this could affect your vision.

The next generation of drugs are the biologic DMARDs. These are genetically engineered versions of natural substances in the body designed to target parts of your immune system that drive inflammation, such as the inflammation-inducing cytokines TNF (tumor necrosis factor) alpha and interleukin-2. Examples are rituximab (Rituxan, MabThera) and abatacept (Orencia). These have much more serious side effects than the conventional DMARDs because they suppress the immune system more actively, increasing the risk of infections and the reactivation of viruses in the body, like chicken pox, which in adults causes shingles. Before starting a biologic, you must be screened for several possible infections that might be lying dormant in your body but could reactivate; for example, tuberculosis and hepatitis B and C. Often, after starting with methotrexate, biologic agents are added once MTX loses its effectiveness. Research shows that this type of combination therapy reduces symptoms and prevents joint deterioration in approximately 50 percent of RA patients.

Yet it is not successful for the remaining 50 percent.[19] As a result, a lot of research has focused on finding another option. The newest are the proteasome inhibitors, a class of drugs that targets an inflammatory compound called NFkB (an acronym for nuclear factor kappa B) and destroys B lymphocyte plasma cells, the immune cells that make antibodies. But it has significant side effects, such as numbness and tingling in your hands and feet, a low white blood cell count, diarrhea, and an increased risk of developing a serious infection. Since other therapies are safer and more effective, this isn't recommended yet for RA or other arthritis conditions.[20]

Clearly, there is a need for better therapy. Even when conventional DMARDs and biologic DMARDs drive the disease into what appears to be remission, low amounts of inflammation remain in the joints—like the part of the iceberg that's under the water—which increases your risk of relapse. Also, some patients don't respond to these medications at all and need another option. The functional medicine approach is that other option. Researchers are now catching on to this and have begun to focus on treating gut bacteria and using probiotics as another way to treat RA. I explain this more in chapter 5, "The Gut-Arthritis Connection."

The Medication Journey: Remission

No matter which approach is used to treat your RA, it is important to know the goals and the criteria to determine if you are in remission and, therefore, when you can stop or taper your treatment. Remission, by the conventional medical definition, means that your arthritis symptoms and/or lab tests have improved enough that they no longer meet the criteria for RA. On one hand, this is great news. But unfortunately, this definition doesn't mean that your inflammation or arthritis is really *gone*. It just means it has dropped below the level of detection as measured by a combination of your symptoms and blood tests.

The most commonly used tool for assessing your symptoms, monitoring your treatment, and deciding if you are in remission is the DAS28. "DAS" stands for disease activity score, which relies on three criteria: (1) a physician's assessment of the number of swollen and tender joints in your hands, wrists, elbows, shoulders, and knees; (2) your overall self-assessment of your symptoms; and (3) a laboratory marker of inflammation (erythrocyte sedimentation rate blood test or C-reactive protein blood test). The score is then calculated from a complicated formula, but, fortunately, it's easy to find an online tool to help with this calculation. The DAS28 score is often used to establish a baseline at your first doctor's visit and followed over time. The only drawback is that you need to have the blood test for the inflammation markers on the day of the examination, and sometimes it's hard to coordinate having your blood drawn on the same day as your physical. DAS28 scores are divided into three levels:

Less than 2.6 is low disease activity;

Between 2.7 and 3.2 is moderate disease activity; and

Between 3.3 and 5.1 is high disease activity.

Clearly, the lower you score, the better.[21] Using the DAS28, remission is defined as a score of less than 2.6, which is minimal pain and normal inflammatory markers. Until you achieve that target, your doctor will continue treating you with different medications. But does this really represent the absence of disease and give you a clean bill of health? The answer is definitely no.

Researchers from the University Clinic of Erlangen-Nuremberg in Germany conducted a randomized controlled study of people in remission based on the DAS28 criteria. In this type of study, patients are randomly assigned to either a group that receives treatment or a control group that doesn't, and they are followed over time. It is considered the most reliable type of study, one reason being that researchers are "blind" to who is getting the treatment and who is not. Their goal was to understand how to know who would be at risk for a relapse when tapering or stopping their medication. While all the study participants met the DAS28 criteria for remission, 33 percent still had rheumatoid arthritis based on the stricter ACR 2010 definition. None of these people had tender or swollen joints, 82.2 percent were on methotrexate, and 40.6 percent were on MTX and a biological DMARD. Some of the patients were left on their current medication, while others were tapered or stopped. The authors looked at the relapse rates for both groups: 15 percent of the subjects who stayed on their full-dose prescription medications relapsed within twelve months, and 44 percent of those who tapered or stopped their treatment relapsed in the same time frame. Clearly, almost half of the people who started tapering weren't *really* ready to do so, pointing out that the conventional definition of remission does not mean the absence of disease. For them, arthritis was just simmering below the surface, waiting to emerge again when medication was stopped.

On the flip side, 56 percent of the study participants who went off their meds remained in remission, a reminder that stopping your medication is truly an achievable goal. The authors found that the ACPA (anti-citrullinated peptide antibody) levels were the main factor in determining the risk for relapse. This makes sense because other studies have shown that high levels of these antibodies were associated with more severe disease and changes in the joints even *before* RA was officially diagnosed. Therefore, the authors concluded, the presence of these antibodies in people whose RA is in remission may reveal an underlying autoimmune process that is still active, which undermines the efforts to stop medication.[22] The take-home message is that if you still have high levels of ACPA, the fires are not out, so this is not the time to go off your medication. The Arthritis Protocol is what you need.

In another study, researchers from the Autonomous University of Barcelona looked at hand MRIs of people with RA who were in remission as defined by the DAS28. Almost 96 percent had ongoing joint inflammation. For me, this is additional confirmation that the DAS28 is not a true measure of the absence of inflammation and shouldn't be used to determine remission. Ninety-six percent is almost everyone! True remission *should* be a total absence of joint inflammation related to RA—meaning zero risk that any joint damage will progress—something found in less than 5 percent of patients in remission.[23] To me, this means that most people with RA who think they are truly in remission when being treated by prescription medication and using conventional remission criteria actually have ongoing oxidative stress and joint inflammation. Left untreated, it will likely progress to more joint damage. This highlights the need for different remission guidelines and a treatment approach that goes beyond targeting what's on the surface and addresses the origin of inflammation so that the fires are extinguished completely. It comes down to redefining the goals of treatment and the disease itself. Doctors should focus on treating oxidative stress and the cause of inflammation, not just suppressing symptoms, which is what conventional medication appears to be doing. We can do better than helping people feel "good enough."

The most important measure is probably how you feel. Your body has an innate intelligence, and if you are paying attention, you *know* that something is or isn't right. (Having some kind of meditation or mindfulness practice can help cultivate your ability to check in with yourself about how you're feeling. Mindfulness just means paying attention to the present moment and not getting lost in thoughts about the past or future. Practice quieting your mind because it will help you notice what's going on in your body in *this* moment.) In medicine, your perspective and the symptoms that you report are called patient-reported outcomes. In the research, it's not clear what this reveals about inflammation and damage, but it makes sense that how a person feels reflects some change in the underlying activity of their disease and this is a good option for following progress—especially when lab tests aren't available. Patient-reported issues related to rheumatoid arthritis include pain, psychological distress, sleep problems and fatigue, and a disruption in their general ability to function and cope at home and work.[24]

Because a change in how you feel is very important, occurs over a short period, and gives us real-time feedback, I closely follow how patients say they feel on the Arthritis Protocol, to make sure we are on the right track. June is a good example of this. Throughout our time together, whenever she had more pain in her hands, her markers of inflammation would go up. But I always knew where she stood just based on her reports about how she felt, and I used this to determine how her treatment was going and when we could taper her prednisone. We decided to try to get her off the corticosteroid even though her CRP level, which had dropped dramatically from where we started, was still mildly elevated.

CHAPTER 2

Spondyloarthritis

Spondyloarthritis is a group of conditions that have inflammation and arthritis of the spine as the central feature. Psoriatic arthritis (PsA) is the most well known, and you've probably seen the countless TV commercials for PsA medications. But this isn't the only inflammatory disorder in the spondyloarthritis family. It also includes AS, juvenile spondyloarthritis, reactive arthritis, and acute anterior uveitis. In addition to affecting the joints the way that other forms of arthritis do, diseases under this umbrella also target the enthesis: the part of a tendon or ligament where it attaches to a bone. To make matters worse, having one of these conditions boosts your risk of inflammatory bowel disease (ulcerative colitis or Crohn's disease) and vice versa. Let's focus here on the two most common forms of spondyloarthritis, PsA and AS.

Psoriatic Arthritis (PsA)

PsA, which affects 2 percent to 3 percent of the population, typically involves the larger joints, especially the spine, unlike rheumatoid arthritis, which does not. PsA can also turn up in various parts of the body, including the fingers and toes. People with eye inflammation such as uveitis and iritis are more likely to have PsA and vice versa. Psoriatic arthritis affects men and women equally. Because there are no specific blood tests or other diagnostic procedures for PsA, a diagnosis is based on a scoring system called CASPAR (see sidebar), which focuses on symptoms that your doctor can see and those that you report.[1]

CLASSIFICATION CRITERIA FOR PSORIATIC ARTHRITIS (CASPAR)

- You have inflammatory arthritis, enthesitis (inflammation of the enthesis in a tendon or ligament), or lumbar (lower back) pain, combined with at least 3 points from the following:
  - You currently have psoriasis: 2 points.
  - You have had psoriasis in the past: I point.
  - You don't have psoriasis, but someone in your immediate family does: I point.
  - Your nail has separated from your nail bed on any finger: I point.
  - You experience inflammation of any finger or toe (current or in history recorded by a rheumatologist): I point.
  - Your blood test is negative for RF: I point.
  - An X-ray shows bone proliferation (not a bone spur) resulting in a fuzzy appearance around the joint: I point.

Imaging may be used to evaluate your joints and make a diagnosis. An X-ray is the typical first step, but an MRI is often the best choice because it is better at picking up damage and swelling in the tendons. An ultrasound is another option, and the newer power Doppler ultrasounds have the potential to look deeper into the joint area, making it an accessible and very useful tool for diagnosing PsA and knowing when there is true remission, with an absence of inflammation.[2]

Psoriasis is a skin condition characterized by red patches covered with silver scales that can appear anywhere on the body. An estimated 20 percent to 30 percent of people who have it also have PsA. If you have arthritis and psoriasis anywhere on your body, even if it is a tiny patch, then you probably have PsA. This is why your doctor must perform a full skin exam, including your scalp and behind your ears. Because psoriasis is thought to be a simple skin condition, many people don't realize that psoriatic arthritis can be very debilitating and brings with it an increased risk of depression, obesity, and metabolic syndrome, a disease defined by too much belly fat that causes high levels of inflammation in the body. These health conditions impair your quality of life and increase your risk of death from any cause.[3] The symptoms of metabolic syndrome include a higher hip-to-waist ratio, high blood pressure, high cholesterol, and either prediabetes (elevated insulin levels or blood sugar) or clinically diagnosed diabetes, where medication is required to control blood sugar.

More than 80 percent of sufferers see skin changes about a decade or more before they actually feel any arthritic pain. Conversely, you can have arthritis for years before seeing any psoriasis, so this skin condition isn't required for diagnosis. Because this can be confusing, a rheumatologist is usually needed to diagnose someone without psoriasis.

There are five subtypes of PsA, as defined by what is known as the Moll and Wright Classification System. Although the categories seem very clear-cut, many people don't fit neatly into one of them, so a diagnosis isn't always obvious. In conventional medicine, deciding which category you are in helps determine your treatment. In functional medicine, the category doesn't matter because inflammation is the underlying cause in all of them, and, just like in RA, an imbalance in the gut is the likely culprit. As a result, the treatment is the same. But I'll detail the five categories here to show that you can have PsA without psoriasis:

- *Asymmetric Arthritis in a Few Joints.* This involves five or fewer medium-large joints, such as one wrist or knee, and usually only on one side of your body. This is different from rheumatoid arthritis, which typically affects both wrists (bilateral, or symmetrical), and the small joints of the hands and feet are affected before the larger joints.

- **Symmetrical Arthritis of Many Joints.** This category resembles RA in two ways: the disease involves multiple small joints on both sides of the body, and up to 50 percent of people with PsA have X-ray evidence of damage to the bone inside the joints. If you have this pattern of arthritis, it is very important that your physician order the blood tests for RA.

- **Distal Interphalangeal Arthritis.** This is arthritis in the last joint in the tips of your toes and fingers. Usually there is also pitting on the nail and a painless separation of the nail from the nail bed. If you don't have psoriasis, this kind of PsA can resemble osteoarthritis, and an X-ray should be able to help your doctor tell the difference.

- **Spondyloarthritis.** This arthritis affects the spine or one or both sacroiliac joints that connect the base of the spine and the pelvis. The lower back pain of spondyloarthritis mirrors that of ankylosing spondylitis, which is why doctors sometimes confuse the two conditions. However, AS can be diagnosed with a genetic blood test called HLA-B27. If the test is negative, you are more likely to have PsA.

- **Arthritis Mutilans.** This severe form, which 20 percent to 40 percent of people with PsA can develop, can cause extreme deformities, bone destruction, and irreversible loss of function. This is a good reminder that, just as with RA, early diagnosis and treatment are important for psoriatic arthritis too.[4]

My patient Robin, a fifty-six-year-old woman happily married with two children, is a good example of someone who didn't fit neatly into any of these categories. When she came to see me, she said that her severe fatigue had been going on for ten years, while the chronic pain in her hands, wrists, knees, elbows, neck, and back started when she was nursing her first baby—fifteen years earlier. At my patients' first visit, I always ask them to rate their pain on a scale of 1 to 10. Robin put hers at a 5. In addition, about two months prior to her seeing me, Robin's left middle finger developed a painful case of stenosing teno-synovitis (better known as trigger finger), in which the finger bends and locks in position. This pattern of arthritis and joint pain doesn't fit any of the above categories, but because Robin had developed psoria-sis in her twenties, I knew she had PsA. This was confirmed by blood tests that showed normal RF, ACPA, CRP, ESR, and ANA, and were negative for Lyme disease and other infections, ruling out any other likely culprit.

Robin's psoriasis started on both of her knees and elbows, with flare-ups that would last about three weeks. When she first came to see me, she was typically getting about three to four outbreaks a year on her scalp and neck and between her breasts, which she was managing with topical steroid creams. Robin controlled her arthritis with over-the-counter pain medication, never needed to take strong prescription medication, and never consulted a rheumatologist for a definitive diagnosis.

As part of my detective work with all new patients, I asked Robin whether she had any digestive symptoms. She told me she often felt gassy and bloated after eating and that she'd experienced two epi-sodes of severe abdominal pain, but her doctors never found the cause. Given her digestive symptoms, in addition to starting her on the Two-Week Jump-Start Leaky Gut Diet, I had her take a stool test to determine the health of her gut bacteria. This test showed sig-nificant bacterial dysbiosis, and after treating the gut with herbs and probiotics, her arthritis improved quickly. I will explain more about dysbiosis and her treatment in part 2, "Heal the Gut, Heal the Joints," as well as the research linking a healthy gut to healthy joints.

Ankylosing Spondylitis (AS)

Although AS is a potentially disabling chronic inflammatory condi-tion, some people have mild forms of the disease. Its main symptoms are severe chronic back pain and stiffness—which makes sense, considering that "ankylosis" means stiffening of a joint, and "spondylos" refers to a vertebra. What happens is that new bone forms between the joints in the spine, creating bony bridges and causing progressive stiffness. If it's not treated early enough in some people, it can result in spinal fusion, where the vertebrae are permanently fused together. Two to three times more men are afflicted with AS than women are.

You are said to have ankylosing spondylitis if you are younger than forty-five and have three features: (1) chronic back pain lasting longer than three months, (2) inflammation of the sacroiliac joints diagnosed by an X-ray or MRI, and (3) a positive genetic test for a protein called HLA-B27. The latter is positive in roughly 90 percent of people with AS. Without all three, it is unlikely that you have this condition, so you and your physician need to keep looking for another diagnosis. If I suspect that a patient has AS, I order the HLA-B27 test; if it's positive, I send him for X-rays or to his rheumatologist to confirm. While it is possible to be diagnosed with AS without a positive HLA-B27 test, it is very uncommon, and therefore if your test is negative, it probably isn't AS.

In people with low back pain, the prevalence of AS is about 4.6 percent to 5 percent. In the United States, it is estimated to be 0.2 percent to 0.5 percent of the population as a whole. Rates of AS vary by ethnicity. Non-Hispanic white people have a 7.5 percent chance of being HLA-B27 positive, which is the highest of all the ethnic groups, and black non-Hispanics have the lowest at 1.1 percent. For people who are HLA-B27 positive, there is a 5 percent to 6 percent rate of getting AS. While these numbers might not seem very high, when you are looking at billions of people, it is a big cause of concern. And while it might seem that there isn't much you can do because of its genetic connection, this is absolutely not the case. Just like with rheumatoid arthritis, finding and treating the triggers for inflammation, wherever they come from, will improve symptoms. Gut health is important for people with AS, too, and we'll talk more about this in part 2, "Heal the Gut, Heal the Joints."

Before we leave the topic of AS, I want to tell you about two of my patients. The first is Sharon, who developed arthritis years after she'd had a severe case of Crohn's disease, an inflammatory disease of the small bowel. She was a very healthy twenty-seven-year-old who ran four miles a day and played competitive soccer. Sharon developed terrible diarrhea after she ate raspberries infected with a certain parasite. Apparently, many people died from this outbreak. She was hospitalized for a week and needed many courses of antibiotics and antiparasitics.

According to Sharon, her gut was never the same, and ever since then, she'd had gas, bloating, and intermittent diarrhea. This is a common story that I hear: a terrible illness changes how you feel even after it is supposedly gone. A few years after the initial illness, Sharon developed worsening symptoms with fever, pain, and diarrhea, and was diagnosed with Crohn's disease. Her doctors made the diagnosis by way of endoscopy—using a thin, flexible fiberoptic scope to look down her throat and into her stomach and small intestine. She was put on an immunomodulator medication called 6-MP (brand name, Purinethol), which made her so tired that she had to quit her job and sleep all the time. But it did help her get healthy enough to become pregnant, and she had her first baby about eight years before she came to see me. Sharon wasn't well, but she was okay. After the birth of her child, she had loose stool with three to four bowel movements daily and lots of nausea and pain in the lower right quadrant of her abdomen.

Sharon felt good enough to stop taking 6-MP, but then her back pain started. It was so severe that she couldn't walk. "The back pain overshadowed my gut problems," she says. After an appointment with a rheumatologist, Sharon learned she was HLA-B27-positive, and X-rays showed sacroiliitis—inflammation of sacroiliac joints—and also arthritis that was affecting almost her whole spine. Based on this combination of symptoms and test results, she was diagnosed with ankylosing spondylitis. She also had some stiffness and tendonitis in her hands, but her severe back pain was the most intense and disabling of her symptoms.

For three years, Sharon tried various medications, including steroids and two biologic immunosuppressants—adalimumab (Humira) for her back pain and infliximab (Remicade) for her Crohn's—but she stopped them because they gave her yeast infections. This can happen when your immune system becomes so suppressed. One time, she went off all the medication, but her Crohn's flared up so severely that she had to be hospitalized, and was given several courses of antibiotics.

Shortly after her hospital visit, Sharon found out she was pregnant again. Although she was thrilled to be having another child, the unplanned pregnancy was very hard on her body. It left her so weak and tired that she needed IV fluids just to get through the nine months. She stayed off her medication but had terrible back pain and anxiety. The Crohn's was never in remission, just simmering along with monthly bouts of watery stool. After Sharon's baby was born, she went on the anti-inflammatory agent mesalamine (Apriso) for her Crohn's. Finally, she was in remission, and she's been on the drug ever since.

For two years after her baby was born, Sharon struggled with back pain until she finally decided she couldn't take it anymore. She started a new immunobiologic called certolizumab (Cimzia), which she'd been on for two years before coming to see me and took in the form of a shot every two weeks. This gave her relief for about ten days, but it would wear off, and then Sharon would be in terrible pain for the remaining four days until her next injection. Even on all her medications, she still suffered from debilitating pain in her back and also in the Achilles tendons that run from the calf down to the heel. This serious discomfort, combined with anxiety and stress, made it hard for her to get through the day, and by the evening, she couldn't function enough to care for her children, who were four and six years old at the time. To sleep at night, Sharon took the anti-anxiety medication lorazepam (Ativan) and a narcotic pain reliever called hydrocodone (Hysingla, Zohydro ER). She was also on duloxetine (Cymbalta), an antidepressant that can help with pain, and pregabalin (Lyrica), for nerve pain she was having down her leg because of a herniated disc.

To say that she was a mess when she arrived at our first appointment is an understatement. I share Sharon's story because I want to make the point that AS can be extremely debilitating, and, for some people, my initial goal with functional medicine is to reduce the pain so that life becomes less overwhelming and more manageable. Sharon is also an example of someone with the classic relationship between inflammatory bowel disease and spondyloarthritis. There has always been a known association between these two health conditions, and it underscores everything that I am sharing in this book: namely the connection between the gut and bodywide inflammation.

I'll share more of Sharon's story and how I treated her in chapter 6, "How to Heal the Gut," but like all my patients with inflammatory arthritis, she followed the Arthritis Protocol. As of this writing, Sharon and I have been working together for one year. Although we are still at the beginning of our work together, her quality of life has improved greatly. She can now run around with her children—something she couldn't do before—she's having normal bowel movements, and, when she takes her prescription medication, Cimzia, it works for the fourteen days until her next dose. These are baby steps, but she is certainly moving in the right direction.

Not everyone with ankylosing spondylitis has a debilitating form like Sharon. Tina, a fifty-two-year-old patient, is a perfect example of someone with a mild form of the disease. For ten years, this Pilates instructor has had AS with mild back pain that she was managing with meloxicam (Mobic), a prescription nonsteroidal anti-inflammatory drug, or NSAID. When she went skiing, she would take extra Mobic to manage her discomfort. Tina came to see me primarily to learn what to eat for better health and to see if she could get off Mobic. After following the Arthritis Protocol, she is now tapering her medication, has no more back pain, and feels more energetic than ever. She knows that AS can potentially be a chronic illness that she will have to manage and live with, but she is committed to preventing it from becoming debilitating. So far, so good.

Conventional Medication

The approach to treating and measuring remission in psoriatic arthritis is similar to rheumatoid arthritis in many ways. However, because PsA does not typically have positive laboratory markers to follow, clinical remission is usually defined as an absence of arthritis symptoms, and this is the goal in people with ankylosing spondylitis as well. Therefore, in contrast to RA, the target for treatment is minimal disease activity.

Nonsteroidal anti-inflammatory drugs and corticosteroids are commonly used to manage both PsA and AS. NSAIDS can be divided into two categories: nonselective and selective. Nonselective NSAIDs, available without a prescription, include aspirin, ibuprofen (Advil, Motrin, and other brands), and naproxen (Aleve). They are more likely to damage your gut—for instance, bringing about gastritis (inflammation in the stomach that can feel like heartburn) and ulcers—and, from a functional medicine perspective, to injure the fragile gut lining and aggravate leaky gut. The selective NSAIDs, a group known as COX-2 inhibitors, are great at relieving pain and less likely to cause gastrointestinal problems. Examples include diclofenac (Voltaren), celecoxib (Celebrex), and indomethacin (Indocin, Tivorbex). However, they increase your risk of heart attack and stroke, so they should be used only for a short amount of time and not if you have heart disease. For treating PsA, NSAIDs are often used with methotrexate.

Just like it is in rheumatoid arthritis, MTX is the foundation of therapy for people with PsA and AS, even though relatively few studies have examined its effectiveness. The available studies concluded that the drug isn't very effective when used at doses of less than 15 milligrams a week and that it works best when combined with a biologic DMARD such as infliximab. DMARDs have opened up a whole new approach to managing PsA successfully. Currently the US Food and Drug Administration (FDA) has approved the following TNF inhibitors for use in psoriatic arthritis: infliximab, adalimumab, certolizumab, etanercept (Enbrel, a TNF blocker), and golimumab (Simponi, a once monthly TNF blocker). Overall, the different drugs seem comparable. That said, sometimes if you don't respond well to one, you may respond well to another. I have seen this happen often. However, there are significant side effects and concerns about long-term use of these drugs, which is why I spent so much time talking about the need to taper and stop these medications as soon as possible.

The newest kids on the block for treating PsA and AS are drugs that specifically target different cells of your immune system. They act like guided missiles at really taking out your immune response in the skin and joints. Many of these are being studied for RA as well. These include Janus kinase (JAK) inhibitors, which block the activity of a family of enzymes, and the genetically engineered monoclonal antibody rituximab. While studies are looking at the use of these medications in large populations of people with PsA, early research results were promising enough that many of these are already in use and available. Each drug has its own side effects, but just like the other biologics, each is a potent immune suppressor and raises the same concern about developing infections and reactivating old viruses such as shingles and mono.

Some older treatments are used in spondyloarthropathies (SpA) that are not used in RA. The first is called sulfasalazine, which is commonly used to treat inflammatory bowel disease. Because IBD is associated with spondyloarthritis, it makes sense that it would be used for people with this type of arthritis. In the limited number of studies that have looked at this drug's effectiveness, it appears that arthritis improves in some people, but sulfasalazine doesn't halt the progression to joint damage. Another DMARD medication, leflunomide, demonstrated better success, with 58.9 percent of people treated showing improvement compared with 29.7 percent of the untreated group. Nevertheless, this drug causes liver toxicity, especially if combined with MTX, and requires careful monitoring.

Another class of drugs are the immunosuppressants. The most commonly used is called cyclosporine, which is marketed under several brand names. Along with tacrolimus (Prograf), cyclosporine is a very strong inhibitor of immune cells called T lymphocytes. Numerous studies have shown that treatment with immunosuppressants improve symptoms of psoriasis and arthritis and that they can be combined with MTX or with a biologic DMARD (TNF inhibitors) for even greater benefit. Cyclosporine and tacrolimus can damage the kidneys, however, and using this drug requires close monitoring.[5]

Whether you have RA, SpA, or any of the other inflammatory arthritis conditions, the goal is always to stop the disease so that you don't have permanent joint damage. While I have shared information on medication, it is critical to note that these drugs don't cure the foundational issues and aren't the only way to stop the disease and induce remission. While they might be necessary to help you back off from the edge of the cliff in times of severe distress, this book offers you the true path to curing the inflammation deep in your joints; to put out the embers so that you will have true remission, not just improved or minimal symptoms. Using this approach makes it quicker and easier to taper off your medicine and reduces the chances of the arthritis coming back.

CHAPTER 3

Osteoarthritis (OA)

Like many people, I thought that osteoarthritis (OA) was the inevitable damage to our joints that came with age, and you couldn't do much about it. I viewed it differently from inflammatory arthritis, which is a group of diseases rooted in the gut. Yet after years of working with patients, I realized that OA is also made worse by inflammation that starts elsewhere in the body, including the gut, and is also influenced and triggered by lifestyle choices such as diet and exercise. Stress and traumatic experiences also have an impact. While writing this book, I encountered an interesting case of OA in a patient who is actually my mother, Barbara. By working with her, I became even more convinced that lifestyle changes to lower inflammation can help treat OA. Here's what happened:

My mother came back from a bucket-list trip to China, a dream vacation that she had loved. On the last day of her trip, she could barely walk because of her knee pain. Being an extremely active and interested seventy-six-year-old, she had spent the three-week trip walking many miles per day and taking part in every possible excursion, such as climbing up and along the Great Wall. When she got home, she was diagnosed with osteoarthritis by an orthopedic specialist. Because my grandfather had both knees replaced when he was in his seventies, and my aunt and uncle have OA in their hands and knees, my mother thought her pain was just par for the course. She assumed she would have to live with it and adjust her life accordingly. For example, she thought she'd have to stop playing golf, like her father had, and limit her travel to bus trips—no more walking tours. Although mothers are usually right, I proved her wrong. After making some important changes to her lifestyle and staying on the program that I gave her, which included an anti-inflammatory diet and supplements (the Arthritis Protocol, which I will show you later), and an exercise plan, my mother was able to pick up her golf clubs and remain active, with no pain. Her story prompted me to catch up on the latest medical research on osteoarthritis—the leading cause of disability worldwide—and confirmed that it is very treatable using the Arthritis Protocol.

In 2015, researchers at the University of Catania in Italy estimated that OA in any joint affected about half of the over-sixty-five population worldwide, with more women affected than men. It also causes more problems with walking and climbing stairs than any other disease. For a long time, OA was viewed as a "wear-and-tear" disease caused by an overload on the joints that eventually destroyed its tissue: first the cartilage and then the bone. Now it has been redefined as a multifactorial disease that is also influenced by lifestyle choices such as diet and exercise, and health conditions like obesity and diabetes.[1] In the United States, OA is the most common form of arthritis, affecting twenty-seven million people, and the third leading cause of years lived with a disability.[2] Also called degenerative arthritis or degenerative joint disease, OA involves the breaking down of protective joint cartilage, which then exposes the bone below to damage. When pain limits how much you move this joint, the muscles around it may begin to atrophy, and the ligaments can become lax. Conventional treatment usually combines pain medication, exercise, and lifestyle changes, but even with these measures, many people opt for joint replacement, since the pain becomes too debilitating and impairs their quality of life.[3]

A scoring system from 0 to 4 based on X-ray findings helps determine if you have OA. The X-ray looks for one or more specific patterns, including a bony outgrowth (called an osteophyte, or bone spur) linked to deteriorating cartilage; narrowing of the space between the joints; an abnormal hardening of joint tissue (called sclerosis); cysts; and deformity. Having an osteophyte gives you a score of 2, which is the minimum needed for an OA diagnosis. Your score goes up if you have any of the additional features such as joint space narrowing, sclerosis, cysts, or deformity. In addition to your score, by measuring and tracking how much the joint space narrows, your doctor can determine whether your arthritis is getting worse. The most common joints affected are the knees, hips, and hands. There is a difference between OA that appears on an X-ray—called radiographic osteoarthritis—and OA that's determined by symptoms, which include pain, aching, or stiffness in the joint. Not everyone with radiographic OA has joint pain, and vice versa. One important note: just because an X-ray reveals that you have arthritis *doesn't mean you have to be in pain*. The pain is triggered by other factors—especially by the presence of inflammation in the body, and that is something we can improve.

Another way to look at the statistics is to measure your lifetime risk of developing symptomatic osteoarthritis. Men have a 40 percent chance and women a 47 percent chance of having symptoms of OA in their knees. Your risk goes up to 60 percent if you have a body mass index (BMI) of 30 or more. (BMI is a measure of body fat based on your weight and height.)[4] A Spanish study of more than three million people found that newly diagnosed OA in the hands is most common between the ages of sixty and sixty-four, whereas that of the hip and knee increases as we get older. Data from the National Health Interview Survey, carried out annually by the CDC, found that the onset of new symptomatic knee OA peaked between ages fifty-five and sixty-four. When young adults develop osteoarthritis, it is typically caused by a prior joint injury; this is known as post-traumatic or secondary OA.[5]

Risk Factors for Osteoarthritis

Putting all the research and information together, obese women over the age of forty-five who have had a previous joint injury are at the highest risk for OA. You can see that the risk factors for OA are very focused on age, obesity (especially having a lot of fat in your abdomen), and injury. This is different from inflammatory arthritis like RA, which has its roots in autoimmunity, immune dysfunction, and gut health. But like inflammatory arthritis, OA is also believed to be caused by environmental triggers like your lifestyle (considered part of your environment)—especially your diet if you are genetically susceptible. From studies of twins, it appears that genetics accounts for about 50 percent to 65 percent of the cause. This number is higher when it comes to OA in the hand and hip than osteoarthritis of the knee. The easiest way to understand your chances of developing OA is to look at risk factors that you *can't* control and those that you *can* control.

Risk factors that you can't control include age (your risk goes up as you get older, and this holds true for all joints), being female (and OA tends to be more severe in women, too), a genetic predisposition, your ethnicity, and the fact that you had a joint injury. Although there is an increase in new diagnoses around the time of a woman's menopause, studies haven't shown a specific link to the hormones estrogen or progesterone. The impact of ethnicity in general is unclear, since the studies are conflicting.

An injury to the joint is one of the strongest risk factors for knee OA and for damaging or tearing the meniscus, which is a thickened, crescent-shaped cartilage pad that covers and protects the top of the tibia (the shin bone). Although repetitive use of a joint doesn't increase your risk as much as an injury, it still has an impact. For example, farmers often develop arthritis in their hips, while middle-aged men whose jobs require carrying, kneeling, or squatting have double the risk of knee OA than the average person does. This increases even more if you're overweight. Studies on athletes are conflicting, but it appears that the highest risk of OA is an injury and not the repetitive use of a joint from, say, running or playing soccer. Finally, some studies suggest that abnormal knee alignment and having one leg that is longer than the other may increase your chances of developing OA.

The good news is that there are plenty of factors you can control. These include building up your muscle strength around a joint, to take the stress off the cartilage and other tissues; being physically active; your occupation; your likelihood of sustaining a joint injury; and whether or not you have the primary risk factors of being obese, having diabetes, and not eating a diet rich in anti-inflammatory and antioxidant foods.[6] Just as obesity boosts your chances of developing osteoarthritis of the knee, losing weight can reduce this risk. Some research on obese elderly people with OA shows that weight loss combined with exercise decreased pain and improved joint function. Other studies link a high BMI when you're eighteen years old with an increased risk of undergoing a total hip replacement later in life.

Your risk for symptomatic OA is a little different than for radiographic OA. Women are more likely to have symptoms than men, and African Americans more than Caucasians. Other controllable risks include: strenuous physical activity, especially activities requiring kneeling, knee bending, squatting, and prolonged standing, and knee injury and trauma. Your X-ray pattern can also predict whether or not you will have symptoms. The higher the number on the 0-to-4 scale and the narrower your joint space increase your chances of having symptoms and influence how severe they will be. Although pain is chronic, it is not constant in 49 percent of people, and instead comes and goes.[7]

Lifestyle

Clearly, increasing age and repetitive use of or injury to a joint, coupled with genetics, can set you up for osteoarthritis. However, there comes a tipping point, when something happens that puts you over the top, and your radiographic-only OA becomes symptomatic. My mother never had an X-ray of her knee before her trip to China, but I have no doubt that evidence of arthritis would have appeared on an X-ray long before she developed the pain. So what caused her symptoms? Two years before her knee pain began, my father, her husband of fifty-six years, died suddenly of a massive stroke. This was an extremely traumatic event, which shook my mother to the core.

The grief and emotional turmoil had an effect on her body, both because of the stress and lack of restful sleep and because her lifestyle habits changed dramatically over the following two years. At first, she was somewhat sedentary and mildly depressed, so she didn't take her dog for the long, leisurely walks that she used to enjoy, and she stopped playing golf. My father never drank and liked home-cooked meals, but after he passed away, my mother didn't feel like cooking just for herself. She went from eating salads, fruit, and lean protein to eating processed foods that she could make quickly and didn't require her to go shopping often. She stopped eating vegetables because she didn't feel like preparing them, and practically lived on gluten-free toast and almond butter. While there is nothing wrong with these foods, it isn't healthy to eat them and nothing else. Dessert, which she ate only occasionally when my father was alive, became a nightly treat when my mother went to her golf club for dinner.

In the second year, my mother joined a group of busy, friendly widows in her retirement community. Almost every night, they went out to dinner, enjoying meals that typically included alcohol (too many Bombay Sapphire gin martinis), bread, and dessert, and very little healthy produce. Although she started playing golf again, my mother didn't resume any other exercise routine. This is what I call "retirement syndrome" and is something I see with many patients. Once they stop working, they let go of the usual rules and structure of their eating, drinking, and exercise. They start sipping wine or cocktails most nights, indulging in unhealthy carbohydrates like bread, crackers, and chips (carbohydrates are one of the three basic macronutrients in the diet; the others are protein and fat), and sugar-laden sweets at all their meals out, and limiting their physical activity. While drinking and being more social probably helped my mother cope with her loss, her new lifestyle was not good for her body.

After doing this for a year and a half, she went on that nineteen-day walking tour of China. Although she had been an avid hiker for the previous seven years, this trip was grueling for her. One day when she walked sixteen thousand steps (she kept track), she said that she "collapsed from the pain" in her left knee. The overuse of her knee combined with the inflammation that was already in her body was the tipping point. In fact, my mother's knee "cried" so much that she had to use a wheelchair at the Hong Kong airport. "I was mortified," she says. "It was awful."

When she came to my house on her way back from China, she hobbled into the room. I took one look at her and saw that the whites of both her eyes were bright red and shiny, and her face and eyes looked puffy and swollen. In addition to the swelling in her knee, these were sure signs that her body was inflamed. I put my mother on the Two-Week Jump-Start Leaky Gut Diet for Arthritis, which is the same one that you will do, and had her meet with our nutritionist at the Blum Center for Health so she could learn how to continue the food plan on her own when she returned home to Florida. I told her not to drink alcohol for at least six weeks and gave her the arthritis supplements, including fish oil and curcumin, that I will share with you in chapter 10, "3-Step Arthritis Protocol and Guide." By the time my mother returned home the following week, she was already walking better, with minimal pain.

Because she had no digestive symptoms, I did not have her start step 2, the Intensive Gut Repair program, and instead decided to wait to see if she improved with the Leaky Gut Diet for Arthritis and the supplements. My mother steadily got better, and after about two months, the pain was gone. She started and continues to follow step 3, the Finish-What-You-Started Six-Month Program and the Healthy Eating Plan as her home base, including an exercise program prescribed by her sports medicine doctor. If she hadn't improved after one month, I would have treated her gut. This story highlights that the biggest triggers for OA are lifestyle related, in the forms of the wrong food, stress, and a lack of exercise, and this is where to start your program. But if you have any gut symptoms at all, or if your joint pain doesn't improve significantly with step 1's Leaky Gut Diet and supplements, you must also treat your gut. Now my mother has occasional flare-ups, but they are always set off by food or stress, and she has a healthy foundation to return to and bring herself back to being pain free. My mother's story shows clearly that her inflammatory diet coupled with a lack of exercise contributed to the painful osteoarthritis in her knee.

Here is how exercise, diet, and obesity interact to determine your risk for OA and where you'll get it. Researchers at the University of Catania in Italy created five categories of risk for osteoarthritis. The lowest category includes people who eat diets rich in nutrients and vitamins, and low in animal fat and processed food, and who are moderately physically active. Activity increases lubrication and synovial fluid, which reduces wear and tear on the cartilage and is healthy for the joints. That said, athletes, who typically get OA in the shoulders, arms, hips, and knees, are at a higher risk because of the forced physical activity, moving sometimes in a way that isn't aligned with the body, puts stress on the joints, and increases direct impact on the joint. On the opposite side of the spectrum, being sedentary increases your risk for OA of the spine and shoulders because of weakening muscles and poor posture. People who use computers and smartphones also fall into this category and have an increased risk of osteoporosis in their hands and wrists. Those who eat diets that lack vital nutrients have an increased risk of OA in *all* their joints. Obese people's excess weight and body fat put them at the highest risk for OA—especially of the spine, hips, knees, and ankles. OA is increasingly being thought of as a systemic disease because it's affected by metabolic issues such as obesity, inflamed fat tissue, and systemic inflammation. To put this in perspective, of all people with osteoarthritis, only 5.1 percent of cases are related to injury, while 24.6 percent are related to excess weight or obesity.[8]

Aging

To better understand exactly what happens in the joints when you get OA, researchers at the University of North Carolina at Chapel Hill have been studying the relationship between aging and OA. They use the term "inflammaging" to refer to age-related inflammation. With each passing birthday, low-grade systemic and local inflammation occur, triggered partly by an age-related increase in visceral (abdominal) fat and decrease in muscle mass. You don't need to be obese for this to happen; aging people naturally accumulate fat and lose muscle. However, muscle loss is another part of the obesity connection. Visceral fat is more inflammatory than the fat in your arms and legs, and plays a special role as an underlying trigger for chronic illness. This metabolic-driven inflammation is called meta-inflammation and is coupled with increased free fatty acids (lipids), hyperglycemia (high blood sugar levels), and oxidative stress. Together these promote destruction of the tissues in and around the joint.

Oxidative stress naturally increases as we age and can negatively affect joints by damaging mitochondria, the little furnaces inside every cell that generate energy to keep the cell alive. Aging mitochondria don't handle free radicals as well, and if they overcome the antioxidant capacity of the cell, the cartilage cells (chondrocytes) can be damaged, and this can contribute to OA.

What is the difference between normal joint aging and OA? During normal aging, the articular cartilage stays intact but becomes thinner, and the density of the healthy cartilage cells decreases evenly throughout the joint. There are no signs of inflammation or thickening of the tissue that lines the joint or any bone thickening around the joints. The main difference with osteoarthritis is that irregularities of the cartilage surface happen in focal areas, and the cartilage cells pile up in clusters near sites of tissue damage, causing the synovial lining to thicken.[9]

Obesity

It is believed that people who are obese or have excess visceral body fat have more oxidative stress throughout their bodies, high blood sugar levels, and issues with the metabolic function of the fat cells, which causes abnormal levels of adipokines: inflammatory compounds released from the fat cells. While obesity is also a risk factor for rheumatoid arthritis, it is considered one of the main triggers for OA. To understand how obesity triggers OA, let's start with oxidative stress. The continuous exposure to free radicals causes the chondrocytes to produce compounds called reactive oxygen species (ROS). These directly damage collagen, the main structural protein component of joint cartilage, and change synovial fluid by making it thinner and less protective. Studies suggest that low levels of vitamin C were associated with a higher risk of knee OA and that increasing your vitamin C intake may keep radiographic knee osteoarthritis and pain from getting worse. Low levels of vitamin K, a nutrient that regulates the mineralization of bone and cartilage, was linked to an increased prevalence of bony outgrowths caused by deteriorating cartilage in the knee and hand and a narrowing of joint space in the hand.

Hyperglycemia is common in people who are obese and have diabetes, and it is associated with developing OA that will continue to get worse. Glucose can attach itself to tissues, which damages the tissues directly and also triggers an inflammatory response. When the cartilage collagen gets covered with glucose (a process called glycation), it reduces the function of the cartilage cells and increases aging and senescence, which is when the cells are very quiet and nonfunctional. This isn't good if you want to have healthy tissues that can repair themselves. This process increases stiffness, and reduces strength of the joint, ultimately leading to OA.

Finally, a word about adipokines, compounds that may be the metabolic link between obesity and OA. An example of an adipokine is leptin, a hormone made by fat cells that has been in the news recently for its role in controlling appetite and supporting your ability to lose body fat. Leptin is also the key player in terms of damage to the joint and development of osteoarthritis, and it has been found to trigger proinflammatory compounds (cytokines), which interfere with the function of the cartilage cells. People who have too much body fat tend to have higher leptin levels.[10]

Research shows that obesity is a metabolic disease that affects every cell in the body, so its connection to OA isn't surprising. Over the past several years, with the enormous amount of emerging research on the gut bacteria, the connection between obesity and gut flora is exploding, too. It makes sense, therefore, that your gut health would also influence the development and progression of OA.

While there isn't a definitive cause-and-effect relationship like the one that exists for inflammatory arthritis conditions, research is beginning to find that the gut plays a role in the metabolic inflammation in some cases of OA.[11] We will talk more about this in part 2, "Heal the Gut, Heal the Joints." Because obesity and diabetes increase your risk of osteoarthritis in the hands and knees, it's clear that this condition doesn't develop just from the added force that extra weight places on the joints. As a result, weight loss programs for people with OA should focus on losing body fat as well as weight, because the fat itself is more likely to be the issue. Getting nutrients and vitamins that reduce oxidative stress, and using a lifestyle program to reduce blood sugar and body fat, should be a central focus to prevent OA, improve joint function, and reduce pain. In fact, two studies showed that osteoarthritic knee pain improved from weight loss related to changes in diet and exercise.[12] The Arthritis Protocol is a lifestyle program that will help you do all these things. I will discuss this further in the treatment section of this chapter.

Conventional Treatment

People with OA are usually treated by an orthopedist, whereas inflammatory arthritis patients are followed by rheumatologists. Because orthopedists are also surgeons, unfortunately, they are not very focused on or knowledgeable about options other than giving cortico-steroid shots for pain management, writing prescriptions for physical therapy and pain medication, and ultimately suggesting surgery. In my experience, corticosteroid shots are perhaps a good temporary fix for pain, but in the long run, they damage the joint and can't be used as a permanent or recurring solution when the pain returns, which it usually does.

OA is typically managed with prescription or over-the-counter medications, which don't halt the progression of the disease and have side effects that make long-term use difficult. (I discussed this in depth in chapter 2 on spondyloarthritis.) Acetaminophen and other popular analgesics (drugs for pain relief, including NSAIDs and nar-cotics) increase your risk of heart disease and internal bleeding and can also damage the liver. Long-term use of systemic NSAIDs, such as celecoxib, diclofenac, ibuprofen, naproxen, and aspirin, to relieve OA symptoms could cause serious adverse events, such as gastro-intestinal bleeding, renal damage, and induction or aggravation of bronchial asthma and cardiovascular complications. Usually, after the orthopedist gives the diagnosis and offers a few of these options, the next step is to seek out additional choices.

Physiatrists, doctors who specialize in rehabilitation and physical medicine, also treat osteoarthritis. I know several great physiatrists who are very hands on in terms of teaching exercises and lifestyle changes. They're also experienced with cutting-edge treatments that use your own stem cells, a cell from which a variety of other cells can develop, or platelet-rich plasma (PRP), blood plasma that has been enriched with platelets. (The plasma is the colorless fluid part of your blood, and platelets are a component of blood involved in clot-ting.) The stem cells or PRP is created from your own blood or tissue and then injected into your joints. These treatments trigger joint tis-sues to repair the damaged bone and cartilage, and, when they work, can really help people feel better. Unfortunately, they don't work all the time and can be very expensive, and so they are not realistic as the main treatment approaches for most people with OA.

Let's look at the conventional treatment options for the average person. Researchers from Leiden University Medical Center in the Netherlands studied the nonsurgical options recommended to patients before their hip or knee replacement surgery. Your body mass index (BMI) is defined as a person's weight in kilograms divided by the square of height in meters (kg/m2). Of the study participants, only 11 percent of those who were overweight (a BMI of 25 to less than 30) and 30 percent of those who were obese (a BMI of 30 or greater) said they received nutrition counseling. A mere 28 percent of orthopedic surgeons said they prescribed nutrition programs to their overweight patients. The most commonly offered nonsurgical treatments were education about osteoarthritis (80 percent), NSAIDs (80 percent), physical therapy (73 percent), and acetaminophen (72 percent). The study authors concluded that combinations of these therapies, especially dietary counseling, should be used more often and could reduce or delay the need for surgery.[13]

Exercise has long been a staple treatment for OA. Physical therapy is commonly prescribed by orthopedic specialists and primary care doctors to help build muscle and stabilize the joints, all in the hopes of reducing pain and improving function. In addition to regular physical therapy sessions, you're also sent home with exercises to do daily on your own. Yet, like my mother, Barbara, most people don't do them consistently or even at all. Many studies over the years have shown that exercise and education programs do improve pain, function, self-efficacy, and participation in home exercise. In South Africa, low-income people often have to wait a long time for both hip replacement and knee replacement surgery. Researchers from the University of Cape Town wanted to find a strategy to help these patients, who suffered severe pain, when surgery might not be possible. Study participants were given a six-week exercise and education program. The latter included pain-neuroscience education, self-management strategies, stress management, and advice about nutrition and the importance of weight loss and an active exercise component. Fifty-three percent of participants reported that the intervention improved their pain, and this improvement was sustained over time. When the authors compared their results with previous studies looking at exercise only, they determined that their group demonstrated greater improvement. And the key to making this happen? The education component.[14] Unfortunately, in this same study, 47 percent of the subjects were not helped by exercise or education alone. I am confident that an intensive anti-inflammatory food and supplement plan, like the one that I offer in this book, would have improved these numbers, and I believe that it is time to add nutrition programs to all treatment programs for OA.

Before talking about food in chapter 7, I want to mention the popular dietary supplements glucosamine and chondroitin, which have been used to alleviate joint pain from osteoarthritis for many years. They are thought to support the process of repair in the joint. Although I also give these supplements to patients in my medical practice, I have found them to be beneficial for only some people. Studies have not proven that they will reduce pain or stop progression of the disease. A recent study from the Rheumatology Department at the Jiménez Díaz Foundation hospital in Madrid, Spain, found that after six months of taking a combination of these two compounds, people with knee OA did not see their pain improve. My point is this: if you have been taking a glucosamine and chondroitin supplement and feel it is helpful, then don't stop. There is no harm in taking it. But statistically speaking, most people won't find it beneficial.

One other supplement deserves mention: undenatured type 2 collagen. Joint tissues such as cartilage and bone are made of a protein called collagen, and collagen destruction is associated with the progression of damage in OA and RA. "Undenatured" means the protein is fully intact and hasn't been destroyed by heat. Some studies have shown that taking 10 milligrams daily of an undenatured type 2 collagen supplement—derived from the cartilage of a chicken or other animal—can reduce the inflammation and pain in osteoarthritis, and even possibly reduce the body's autoimmune reaction to its own cartilage. I have been using this in my practice recently, and although I am still not sure how effective it is, I wanted you to know about it.[15]

I still believe that we should focus on the underlying driving forces that damage joints: namely inflammation and oxidative stress. You will learn more about antioxidants and omega-3 fatty acids, which are not part of conventional treatment, in part 4, "The Blum Center 3-Step Arthritis Protocol."

CHAPTER 4

Other Arthritis Conditions

Undifferentiated Arthritis (UA)

The names that are given to different kinds of arthritis can be very confusing, and I want to explain a little more about undifferentiated arthritis. It is considered undifferentiated because the arthritis is at such an early stage that it hasn't turned into full-blown rheumatoid arthritis, psoriatic arthritis, or an autoimmune arthritis such as Sjögren's or lupus. Therefore, no diagnosis can be made other than that you have some form of arthritis that appears to be inflammatory. "Undifferentiated arthritis" is used to describe people who have had arthritis for six to twelve weeks but still don't meet the criteria for any other arthritis diagnosis. This is an important category because 30 percent of people who go to their doctor with early arthritis will initially be diagnosed with UA. Of those, about 30 percent will end up with RA. The other 70 percent will end up with an assortment of diagnoses, including OA and autoimmune diseases.[1]

Initially, Rob, a sixty-year-old attorney, came to see me because his cardiologist prescribed Crestor, and he didn't want to take it. He felt that there had to be a way to control his cholesterol without this medication. But Rob was concerned because his father had undergone a quadruple bypass in his early fifties, which put Rob at a higher-than-average risk of cardiovascular disease. Also, over the course of five years, Rob had gone from 155 to 165 pounds, and the 10-pound weight gain made him feel too heavy.

A family history of prostate cancer also had Rob worried, as his two grandfathers and a cousin had been diagnosed with the disease. Men his age are screened annually with a lab test that measures the blood level of prostate-specific antigen (PSA), a protein produced by the prostate gland. Rob's PSA level had fluctuated greatly over the past ten years. However, all of his prostate exams had been normal, and he was always told that his elevated PSA level reflected not cancer but merely benign prostatic hypertrophy (BPH)—an enlarged prostate. Rob's current plan with his doctors was to watch and wait, and he also underwent an annual ultrasound scan.

The more I talked to Rob, the more I learned about him. Although he slept seven hours a night, he drank two to three cups of coffee every day to stay focused. This could indicate that his quality of sleep wasn't very high, even though the quantity was pretty good. Stress was also an issue. Five years earlier, he had gone through a divorce that had been preceded by two intense, difficult years. It was after this stressful time that his cholesterol and weight started rising. More recently, he had been caring for his aging parents. When I first saw him, Rob had no digestive symptoms of any kind. However, he did tell me that, according to his parents, he'd had celiac disease when he was younger but outgrew it. Celiac is an autoimmune disease triggered by eating gluten, a protein found in wheat, kamut, spelt, barley, and rye, where the immune system attacks and damages the small intestine. Also, by age sixteen, he'd developed an ulcer (a break in the lining of the stomach) and gastritis (inflammation in the lining of the stomach). Rob told me he believed he got these in his stomach because that's where he holds all his stress. This is a story that I hear a lot, especially from people who tend to internalize anxiety.

To help Rob lose those extra ten pounds, I started him on a detox program that included both a food plan and supplements to help increase his liver's ability to eliminate toxins. This is especially effective for losing fat, because toxins are stored in your fat cells; also, reducing your body fat can help lower your cholesterol. Rob also followed an elimination diet similar to what you will do in the Arthritis Protocol. Over the next year, Rob lost eight pounds and lowered his cholesterol enough so that he didn't need medication, thanks to the exercise program he'd started as well as taking fish oil and fiber supplements. Rob followed his treatment plan diligently, and his health appeared to be improving. That was until he developed arthritis seemingly out of the clear blue.

When he sat down in my office, he was very upset and concerned that for the past two months, he'd experienced pain and swelling in the pointer fingers on both hands. He had seen an orthopedist, who took X-rays and assured him there was no damage or any other issues in the joints. Regardless, Rob couldn't bend his fingers, and even taking Aleve did little to help with the swelling and pain. This is where good medical detective work is important. As we talked about what was going on in his life, Rob told me that he was having a hard time selling his apartment, which was affecting him financially. It was also affecting him emotionally because it was preventing him from moving on with his life and moving forward in his relationship with his girlfriend. As if he didn't have enough on his plate, his father was very sick. Because Rob was so stressed, he was not really sticking to the food plan and was eating gluten again.

I sent him home with the Leaky Gut Diet for Arthritis, increased his fish oil supplements, and added an anti-inflammatory curcumin supplement for the arthritis. Curcumin is a compound found in the herb turmeric, which is a type of ginger. It has been shown to inhibit enzymes in the body that cause inflammation. I also had him take home a stool test kit so that I could see what was going on in his gut and to figure out what kind of arthritis he had. I ordered all the blood tests, including rheumatoid factor, anti-citrullinated peptide antibody, erythrocyte sedimentation rate, and C-reactive protein (all of these tests would help me diagnose RA), anti-nuclear antibody, and Sjögren's antibodies (both of these tests would help me determine if he had arthritis from a rheumatic disease). All of his lab tests came back normal, so I diagnosed him with undifferentiated inflammatory arthritis.

Four months later, Rob returned, thrilled that his pain and swelling were 25 percent better, and he was able to use his fingers again. Even though the arthritis wasn't completely gone, the food plan, anti-inflammatory herbs, and increased amounts of fish oil had really helped him. As I mentioned before, when it comes to functional medicine, the type of arthritis a person has—or whether or not he or she has been definitively diagnosed at all—doesn't really matter because the Arthritis Protocol treats all inflammatory arthritis with the same approach.

Also, when I looked at the results of Rob's stool test, it all made sense to me. His gut was infected with a lot of *Candida* and *Rhodotorula*, two different kinds of yeast that can cause dysbiosis by overgrowing in large amounts in the gut, triggering systemic inflammation and arthritis. We began a treatment plan that included herbs and a prescription antifungal medication called fluconazole (brand name, Diflucan). In six months, his arthritis was gone. I will tell you about his exact treatment program in chapter 6, "How to Heal the Gut."

Arthritis from Rheumatic Diseases

Arthritis is a symptom that people often have as part of another auto-immune disease, especially systemic lupus erythematosus, Sjögren's syndrome, and systemic sclerosis (scleroderma). These are called systemic autoimmune diseases because the affected tissues are spread throughout the body instead of being restricted to one particular organ, like we see in an autoimmune disease such as Hashimoto's thyroiditis, for example, which is called an organ-specific autoimmune disease. In contrast to rheumatoid arthritis, these disorders have other systemic features, such as rashes, dry mouth and eyes, muscle pain, and kidney involvement. And so, while the joints may be involved, it is just one of many symptoms. People with RA usually test positive for inflammation, whereas in this group of autoimmune diseases, these tests are often normal or only mildly elevated. Additionally, the typical findings of morning stiffness, symmetric arthritis, and deformities that we usually see in rheumatoid arthritis are not present. The bottom line is that if you have arthritis, it is important to see your doctor to determine if your primary problem is a systemic autoimmune disease or inflammatory arthritis.

Systemic autoimmune diseases all share a common positive test called an anti-nuclear antibody, or ANA. Typically, this is the first test performed because it is extremely rare to have one of these conditions without a positive ANA. If the result is positive, then your doctor can continue to dig deeper and test for specific markers for these conditions. (See the sidebar below for a list of specific tests.) Keep in mind that it is possible to have a positive ANA from a virus such as Epstein-Barr, the virus that causes mononucleosis, and which can continue to cause severe fatigue long after you think the mono is over. You can also get a positive ANA from a bacterium like the tick-borne *Borrelia burgdorferi*, which causes Lyme disease, so a positive result doesn't necessarily mean you definitely have lupus or one of these other autoimmune diseases. For example, a lupus diagnosis hinges on testing positive for ANA as well as for the anti-double-stranded DNA (dsDNA) antibody.

AUTOIMMUNE LABORATORY TESTING

- General screening test: anti-nuclear antibody blood test.
- Systemic lupus erythematosus: anti-double-stranded DNA blood test, anti-Smith (anti-sm, a protein found in the nucleus of a cell) antibody blood test.
- Sjögren's syndrome: anti-SSA and anti-SSB antibody blood tests.
- Systemic sclerosis/scleroderma: scleroderma antibody (Scl-70) blood test, anti-centromere antibody (ACA) blood test, anti-RNA polymerase III antibody blood test.
- Dermatomyositis and polymyositis: creatine kinase and aldolase blood tests; anti-Ro/SSA, anti-La/SSB anti-RNP, anti-Sm, and anti-Jo-1 antibody blood tests.
- Mixed connective tissue disease: anti-U1 RNP antibody blood test.

Because people with all of these systemic autoimmune diseases can have arthritis as part of their condition, it can be challenging for your doctor to determine if you have a purely arthritic condition or an autoimmune disease. For example, lupus is an autoimmune attack that can affect every organ in your body, which is why it can be so devastating. Arthritis and arthralgias (joint pain without inflammation) occur in more than 90 percent of lupus patients and are often some of the earliest manifestations.[2] In systemic autoimmune conditions, the arthritis can be in multiple joints, the way it is in rheumatoid arthritis, but it usually does not cause erosion or deformities. (Although this can occur sometimes, and when it does, the clinical picture can resemble that of RA.) In someone with SLE, erosive arthritis can be predicted by the development of a positive ACPA test.[3] However, conventional therapy still focuses on treating the lupus even though you might develop arthritis. Having this overlap of positive tests for two autoimmune diseases is common, and when I see a lupus sufferer with joint involvement, it just reinforces my resolve to repair the gut bacteria because I know that there is an issue that is amplifying the SLE symptoms. Of course, everyone with autoimmune disease needs to repair his or her gut, but once there is arthritis, that should become the focus.

Sjögren's syndrome (SS) affects exocrine glands throughout the body: organs that secrete fluids, such as the salivary glands in your mouth and the tear-producing lacrimal glands. Dysfunction in these particular glands causes dry mouth and dry eyes, respectively, but Sjögren's sufferers may also experience vaginal dryness and reduced lubrication in the skin and respiratory tract. About 50 percent of people with primary SS have joint involvement, including the synovitis and bone erosion that is seen commonly in rheumatoid arthritis. In fact, patients often start out with Sjögren's, progress to testing positive for rheumatoid factor or the anti-citrullinated peptide antibody, and end up with RA.[4]

Scleroderma refers to thickened, hardened skin. When it involves internal organs, it is called systemic sclerosis. This is an autoimmune disease where not only is the skin affected, but also patients complain of fatigue, swollen hands, and muscle and joint pain. However, the joints usually do not exhibit swelling, and X-rays do not typically show synovitis or bone erosion. In the rare instances when inflammatory arthritis does arise, it often follows a pattern similar to that in RA, called an "overlap syndrome." This is where it seems like you have both conditions going on at the same time. Scleroderma is diagnosed by blood tests, specifically anti-Scl-70, anti-centromere antibody (ACA), and anti-RNA polymerase III antibody. If any of these come back positive, it is likely that this is the underlying condition.

Dermatomyositis and polymyositis are inflammatory conditions affecting the muscles, and their primary symptoms are muscle weakness and pain, with the joints rarely involved. When the skin is affected, the diagnosis is dermatomyositis. Because they are part of the grouping of systemic rheumatic diseases, I am including them here just for your information. Finally, mixed connective tissue disease (MCTD) is a diagnosis given to people who have overlapping symptoms of lupus, systemic sclerosis, and polymyositis. A diagnosis is made because they have a high concentration of a distinct antibody called anti-U1-ribonucleoprotein (RNP). Most people with MCTD will end up with one of the three overlapping conditions years later. A confirmed diagnosis of MCTD requires a positive blood test, but you also need to have the clinical picture of joint pain, muscle pain, and fatigue.

As you can see, the symptoms for all these conditions can overlap, which can be confusing. Nevertheless, there are blood tests to determine if you have one of these. If all the blood tests are normal, and you have persistent inflammatory arthritis for more than eight weeks, you probably have either rheumatoid arthritis, early RA, spondyloarthritis, or undifferentiated arthritis. But even if your health care provider isn't sure exactly which type of arthritis you have, you still have an inflammatory arthritis, and following the Arthritis Protocol will help you feel better.

Arthritis from Infections

Before leaving this chapter, I want to discuss briefly how you can get arthritis from infections, which is very different from inflammatory arthritis or osteoarthritis. This is also different from when the bacterium *Proteus mirabilis* or *Mycoplasma* elicits a reaction in the body that ultimately triggers RA or another inflammatory arthritis. In this case, an actual microbe infiltrates the joint, causing the arthritis. Of all the types of arthritis mentioned in this book, arthritis from infections is the only category where the first line of attack is to treat the infection and not the gut. However, since 70 percent of your immune system lives in the gut, a healthy gut is critical to clear your infection and recover completely. Also, if your doctor prescribes antibiotics, you must take probiotics to protect its damaging effect on good gut bacteria.

Bacteria

Several different kinds of infections can bring about arthritis, including bacteria, viruses, and fungal infection. Bacterial arthritis can cause something called a septic joint. This is usually easy to diagnose because the joint becomes suddenly painful, with the classic signs of infection, including redness, swelling, tenderness, and difficulty moving the joint. Typically, you also develop a fever, which can be very high. The knee is the most common area infected, but other joints that can get infected are the hip, shoulder, wrist, and ankle. Because it's very unusual for it to affect your fingers, it is relatively easy to differentiate bacterial arthritis from rheumatoid arthritis. Moreover, there is usually fluid inside the joint, which your doctor can drain with a needle and send to a lab to identify the bacteria. While these cultures are positive in only one-third of the cases, the blood can be cultured too, and this tests positive in up to 60 percent of adults.

With septic arthritis, the bacteria enter the joint after traveling through the blood, which is why the joint infection usually comes after an infection begins somewhere else. For example, a joint can develop a staph infection after an injury allows this bacterium into your body through the skin. Another test looks for the bacteria DNA in the joint fluid. The most common bugs are the *Yersinia* species, *Chlamydia* species, *Mycoplasma hominis*, *Ureaplasma* species, *Borrelia burgdorferi* (Lyme), and *Neisseria gonorrhoeae*. And sometimes, if an infection such as *Mycoplasma* goes undetected and untreated, it can become a trigger for RA. The most important thing to keep in mind is that if you experience sudden pain in a large joint such as your knees or hips, accompanied by a fever, see your doctor because you might have an infected joint that needs treatment with antibiotics.

In *chronic* infectious arthritis, a bacterium initially causes a mild infection that becomes chronic when left untreated. Common organisms for this kind of arthritis include *Treponema pallidum* (the culprit behind the sexually transmitted disease syphilis, among others), *Mycobacterium tuberculosis* and *Mycobacterium leprae* (which cause tuberculosis and leprosy, respectively), and *Brucella* (a bacterium from unpasteurized milk products), and these infections are commonly found worldwide. Different fungi can also be involved, including *Candida*, *Blastomyces*, and *Coccidioides*, all found in the United States. These fungal infections can occur after a trauma that penetrates the skin, letting the organisms into the body. The difference between these kinds of chronic infections and inflammatory arthritis is that chronic infections usually affect just one joint. They can be identified from a culture of the joint fluid and treated with antibiotics.

Virus

Getting arthritis after having a virus is relatively common. Rubella (caused by the rubella virus), fifth disease (caused by parvovirus B19), mumps (caused by the mumps virus), and hepatitis B (caused by the hepatitis B virus) are the most common viruses, especially in the United States, and simple blood tests can uncover them. Less common are lymphocytic choriomeningitis virus (you would develop meningitis too, an inflammation of the protective membranes covering the brain and spinal cord) and mosquito-borne infections such as chikungunya (East Africa, India), o'nyong-nyong (East Africa), Ockelbo agent (Sweden), Ross River agent (Australia), and Barmah Forest virus (Australia).

Viral arthritis, which is easy to diagnose with a simple blood test, is almost always accompanied by symptoms in addition to joint pain. With rubella and parvovirus, there is usually a rash and fever. Mumps causes fever, headache, and swelling of the parotid glands, which are located on each side of your face, in front of your ears. Hepatitis B can cause arthritis in up to 20 percent of people, as well as urticaria (or hives, with red, raised plaques and itching) and jaundice (yellow skin and yellowing of the white part of your eyes). Arthritis from a virus should last no more than six to eight weeks. If it goes on longer than two months, another diagnosis should be considered. Also, keep in mind that you can have *both* inflammatory arthritis such as rheumatoid arthritis *and* a virus, and it is the virus that might be responsible for a flare-up of symptoms. This is important to know so that you can wait out the virus for those six to eight weeks instead of increasing the dose of your RA medication.[5]

PART 2

Heal the Gut, Heal the Joints

While all four parts of this book are equally important, the relationship between your gut health and joint inflammation is probably the most exciting. Emerging research about the gut microbiome is triggering a revolution in terms of how we understand the gut's role when it comes to systemwide inflammation, especially in arthritis. Here I will share the science and stories of my patients that will illustrate how I use this information in my medical practice to help them—so that I can help you, too.

CHAPTER 5

The Gut-Arthritis Connection

From a conventional point of view, it is very important to know what kind of arthritis you have because each responds differently to medication and varies in its aggressiveness. However, from a functional medicine perspective, the root of inflammation in all inflammatory arthritis conditions is the gut. Although osteoarthritis is technically not a form of inflammatory arthritis, oxidative stress and inflammation are big parts of the problem and causes of pain, and recent research is showing a connection to the gut, too. Thus, treating the gut will improve symptoms from this condition. However, we will focus more on OA in part 3, "Treating Your Terrain," where we will look at the impact of diet and stress on inflammation.

Since the publication of my last book, strong evidence has emerged about the connection between arthritis, gut microbial dysbiosis, and increased intestinal permeability—a condition called leaky gut syndrome. This chapter will explain what this is and how it can trigger arthritis.

The gut bacteria are the collection of microbes that live in the small and large intestine. Every day, it seems that there is more news about their influence on our overall health. This makes sense, since, as I mentioned earlier, 70 percent of your immune system lives just below the intestinal lining—lying in wait to protect you from danger—and has a close relationship with your gut flora. I will show you how imbalanced gut bacteria, a condition called dysbiosis, could be one of the underlying causes of a damaged immune system, bodywide inflammation, and could set the stage for arthritis to emerge. Before digging into the research on this subject, let me explain some fundamentals about your digestive system and why the bacteria in the gut are so important. This will make it easier to understand what can go wrong and how to treat it.

Your Intestinal Lining

The word "gut" refers to your digestive system, or gastrointestinal tract, a long tube that stretches from your mouth to your anus and has the estimated surface area of a tennis court! Given its size, this is your largest daily exposure to potential toxins and infectious organisms that are carried into the body by food you eat or anything else that goes in your mouth. Your stomach is the first line of defense in protecting you. It is the sterilizer, with a pH of 1.5, ready to kill living things that you might ingest accidentally—or, if you love sushi, on purpose. (There are all sorts of microbes in the flesh of animals and fish, and your stomach health is very important if you eat, for example, sushi.) Taking antacids or proton pump inhibitors lowers your stomach acid and increases the possibility that living organisms can make their way past your stomach and into the next part of your digestive system, which is your intestines.

The small and large intestines are tubes lined with a layer of epithelial cells referred to as the intestinal lining, and the cavity of the hollow tube is called the lumen. The ileocecal valve marks the transition from the small intestine to the large intestine, or colon. At approximately twenty-three feet, the small intestine is longer and narrower than the large intestine, which is about five feet long and three inches in diameter. The small intestine has three sections: the duodenum, the jejunum, and the ileum. Digestion occurs mainly in the duodenum. Then all your nutrients are absorbed in the jejunum and ileum, which are lined with villi: fingerlike projections that increase

68

the surface area for absorption and digestion. In contrast, the surface of the large intestine is flat. Its main role is to absorb water and eliminate anything that's not digested, such as the carbohydrate cellulose found in grasses. The colon is also the main reservoir for trillions of good bacteria. The epithelial cells, which are constantly being renewed and released into the lumen to be eliminated as part of stool after living for five days, are part of the intestinal lining. This fragile membrane also includes the blood supply, lymphatics (a network of vessels that are part of your normal circulation like arteries and veins, through which the body's fluids drain from cells and tissues and into the bloodstream), nervous system, and developing immune cells, concentrated in areas called Peyer's patches.

Goblet cells are specialized cells in the intestinal lining that make mucus, and the number of them increases as food passes through the GI tract. This mucus is critical to maintain the gut lining barrier and to prevent good bacteria from mingling with the epithelial and immune cells, which could potentially trigger an immune and inflammatory reaction. The mucous layer is thickest in the colon, where the highest concentration of bacteria live. It also has an inner dense layer that provides a secure physical barrier and contains compounds that are toxic to many bacteria, and a loose outer mucous layer containing nutrients that support the healthy growth of the beneficial flora. Many bacteria live there. Clearly, problems with mucus could increase the risk of damage to the intestinal lining and inflammation because it would allow good bacteria to reach the surface of the colon, and this appears to be associated also with an increased risk of colitis (inflammation in the lining of the colon) and colon cancer.[1]

Leaky Gut

The intestinal barrier covers a surface area of 4,300 square feet and requires 40 percent of your body's energy expenditure to keep it functioning properly. Since the 1980s, almost three thousand published studies have covered the topic of increased intestinal permeability, or leaky gut. Obviously, there is a lot of interest, and for good reason. We now know there is a link between a leaky gut and almost every chronic inflammatory health condition. But what causes it and how? Current research is focused on the intestinal microbiome and conditions of imbalance in the types of gut bacteria as triggers for changes in permeability.

As I mentioned, the barrier of the intestinal lining is composed of epithelial cells, the antimicrobial compounds they make, and a mucous layer. The epithelial cells are attached to one another by what are called tight junctions, which are made of proteins and prevent anything inside the intestine from gaining entry into the body. When these tight junctions are damaged, the result is a leaky gut, or increased intestinal permeability, which means that bacteria, for example, can freely pass through the intestinal lining and into the body, triggering an immune response. This can lead to inflammation throughout the body, resulting in allergies, diabetes, obesity, heart disease, arthritis, and cognitive defects, like memory issues. Even when there is no specific disease, damage to the tight junctions can cause fatigue, difficulty concentrating, and puffiness, which compose the symptoms of what is often referred to as leaky gut syndrome.

Tight junctions are very dynamic and adaptable, and are important regulation points in the epithelial cell lining. They selectively allow into the body ions (molecules with an electric charge) and small water-soluble compounds from the end products of digestion. Several studies suggest that increased intestinal permeability in people with rheumatoid arthritis is related to damage to the tight junctions and increased activity of a protein called zonulin, which allows the passage of antigens into the body. An antigen is a toxin, microbe, food protein, or other foreign substance that causes an immune response in the body, especially the production of antibodies. The immune reactions that this can cause can target the joints.

Keep in mind that just as zonulin allows antigens to pass through, it also opens the gates for immune cells, whose job it is to apprehend and destroy the intruders. The flow goes in both directions, with immune cells flowing out and microbes and other contents of the gut lumen flowing in. Think of it as a wall with small, open gaps that have not been sealed. Interestingly, people with autoimmune disease have higher-than-average levels of zonulin in their blood.

According to a study from the University of Maryland School of Medicine, both gluten and gut bacteria can trigger the release of zonulin and increase intestinal permeability. While harmful bacteria had this effect, the researchers found that good bacteria could do the same if they came in direct contact with the cells on the surface of the small intestine, which under normal circumstances is prevented by the layer of mucus lining your gut. Gliadin, a protein found in gluten, binds and releases zonulin. This reaction is very severe in people with celiac disease, but it also affects those without celiac. The study also revealed that tight junctions could be compromised by exposure to two of the primary treatments for many forms of cancer—radiation therapy and chemotherapy—as well as toxins. The researchers call this mechanism for developing a leaky gut zonulin-dependent tight-junction dysfunction, and this appears to happen in both rheumatoid arthritis and ankylosing spondylitis.[2]

More and more evidence suggests that autoimmune diseases are caused by changes in tight junctions in people who are genetically susceptible. One theory is that this group of people are more likely to have a zonulin system that overreacts to an antigen presented in the GI tract, so when it is exposed to a trigger such as gluten, bacteria, or toxins, there is increased intestinal permeability. This then allows the antigen to be sensed by the immune system, triggering an inflammatory and autoimmune response.[3]

Researchers at the Technion-Israel Institute of Technology in Haifa found that tight junction dysfunction is the first thing that triggers inflammatory joint diseases, including rheumatoid arthritis, psoriatic arthritis, ankylosing spondylitis, and juvenile rheumatoid arthritis, and that losing the protection of the mucosal barrier helps these autoimmune and systemic inflammatory diseases develop. They also found that tight junctions are regulated by many factors, including bacteria, yeast, free radicals, enzymes, and other components of the nervous system, the digestive system, and immunity. Many of these factors are regulated by the gut bacteria, which again highlights the importance of having a healthy gut stocked with "good" bacteria. However, over the last fifty years we've learned that many dietary changes appear to be damaging to tight junctions. These include sugar, salt, emulsifiers, and surfactants added to processed food; organic solvents such as alcohol, ethanol, and acetaldehyde; and nanoparticles used to increase absorption of drugs and enzymes released from gut microbes. The results of their research also supported the findings that gliadin in gluten damages the tight junctions.[4] Given the growing evidence that increased permeability brings about arthritis, it seems logical that fixing leaky gut can cure the root cause of the arthritis and reverse the disease. I have seen this repeatedly in the last fifteen years of practicing functional medicine.

Leaky gut can also result from gaps in the epithelial cell lining. The intestinal epithelium is renewed every five days under normal conditions. However, inflammatory molecules released by immune cells or epithelial cells can increase this rate of cell shedding. If the cell turnover outpaces the production of new cells, the result can be holes that aren't plugged up fast enough and, in turn, increased permeability. Keep in mind that the flow goes in both directions, with immune cells flowing out and microbes and other contents of the gut lumen flowing in. Think of it like small open areas along a wall with incomplete sealing of the gaps.[5]

Your diet and any nutrient deficiencies can have an impact on the intestinal barrier. Studies tell us consistently that diets high in fat and processed carbs boost your chances of developing a leaky gut. Fructose, the simple sugar found in fruit but also used as an additive in processed foods, is associated with intestinal bacterial overgrowth and leaky gut. Deficiencies in vitamins A and D also impair the intestinal barrier, change the bacteria, and increase intestinal permeability. On the other hand, quercetin, a flavonoid (a compound found in fruits and vegetables that has antioxidant and anti-inflammatory properties) that is plentiful in grapes and onions, was found to reduce the risk of mucosal damage.[6]

There are many ways that your healthy flora keeps these tight junctions and the barrier working properly. Your good bacteria make nutrients that feed the epithelial cells and help them turn out compounds that increase the production of a protein that strengthens the barrier, according to research from Albert Einstein College of Medicine, in New York. Given the hundred trillion bacteria in the gut, this is a huge number for your immune system to manage. Furthermore, the levels of compounds they secrete, such as by-products of bacteria metabolism and specific chemicals, are enormous. In general, the way the cells in your body communicate with one another is through signaling molecules released by one cell and then received by another. This is true in the gut as well, but in this case, the bacteria release the compounds that are received by the cells in your body, triggering a response in the cells in your gut lining. Research shows a direct chemical communication between the good gut flora and a specific receptor involved in the health of the intestinal mucosa, called toll-like receptors (TLRs). These critical regulators of intestinal barrier function and inflammation have a direct effect on the tight junctions. This research supports the treatment approach we are using, which focuses on restoring robust amounts of good flora to improve the gut environment to both reduce inflammation and reverse and treat leaky gut syndrome.[7]

Your Microbiome

Your gut microbiome is a diverse community of microorganisms that includes bacteria, viruses, and fungi. Bacteria are the most abundant, but the viruses and fungi influence health and disease in ways that we don't quite understand yet. An array of recent research has focused on understanding the role of the bacteria in human health, and this is what I will discuss here.

However, I don't want to diminish the role of yeast in triggering dysbiosis and systemic inflammation. A yeast called *Candida* is sometimes found in the stool of my patients, who always ask where it came from. Just like a garden naturally has weeds, the gut naturally has small amounts of these yeasts. Your body keeps them in check, thanks to the activity of good bacteria, a well-functioning intestinal barrier, and a strong and balanced gut-immune system. Therefore, even though tiny amounts of yeast exist, they cause a problem only if the gut is out of balance, which lets them grow. The herbs that I use in step 2, the Two-Month Intensive Gut Repair, kill yeast as well as bacteria, so if you do have yeast overgrowth, this will be treated as part of this program. But for now, back to the bacteria.

The human intestine harbors an estimated hundred trillion microbes, and even though there are up to an estimated thousand different species of bacteria, only about a hundred of them make up 99 percent of the population. The number of bacteria progressively increases farther down the small intestine, and they also begin shifting from aerobic (meaning they thrive in the air) to anaerobic (meaning they die in the air). In the colon, it is mostly anaerobes, and you can get a sense of how many bacteria are in there when you realize that your feces are 60 percent bacteria! With recent advances in our ability to easily read the genes of different organisms, we can identify all these bacteria instead of relying only on what grew out in culture. According to a 2016 study published in the medical journal *Digestion*, greater bacterial diversity seemed to correspond with better nutritional intake and greater overall health in a group of elderly people.[8] It has been widely cited that there are ten times as many bacteria in our body as human cells. Yet when researchers from the Weizmann Institute of Science in Rehovot, Israel, studied this, they found that the numbers of bacteria and cells were actually equal.[9] Of course, that is still a lot of bacteria!

What influences the health of your flora? Antibiotics can destroy the good bacteria in the gut, and evidence suggests that the gut bacteria may never fully recover after even one course of treatment. Your early life after birth is also important, and it appears that babies inherit their microbiota from their mother during labor, as they pass through the birth canal in the vagina. Studies have shown that babies born by Cesarean section—removed surgically from the womb—have a delay of gut colonization. At six months of age, they have less of the bacteria *Bacteroides fragilis* and *Clostridia* than children born vaginally. These differences in microbiota, still present even seven years later, are associated with an above-average risk of developing type 1 diabetes and allergic diseases such as asthma and food allergies.[10]

Let's review a little background on the names of the gut bacteria before moving on. Every bacteria has a very specific species name, such as *Lactobacillus acidophilus*. But these same bacteria are sometimes referred to in general as *Lactobacillus* spp. When referred to this way, the authors are talking about all the different lactobacillus strains collectively, as a group. To make matters even more confusing, lactobacilli belong to a larger family (referred to as a phylum), Firmicutes. A phylum is like an extended family that includes many, many cousins, and studies that analyze changes in the gut bacteria due to dietary modifications often just refer to these general categories.

Other names you will see frequently are the *Bifidobacterium* species, which belongs to the phylum Actinobacteria. Bacteroidetes is a large family of bacteria that includes the *Bacteroides* and *Prevotella*, two species that are often cited in studies looking at rheumatoid arthritis and the gut microbiome. In general, all these bacteria belong to a phylum that is considered good for us, but you will see that even some of these good bacteria can create harmful environments in the gut if they overgrow, especially if one species increases at the expense of another.

As an adult, the composition of your gut microbiota is related most strongly to your diet, and we will explore this in more detail in chapter 7, "Food and Fire." By and large, people who eat a diet high in animal fat and protein have a pattern of gut flora that is dominated by the *Bacteroides*, while the gut flora of those who consume lots of vegetables and fiber and little animal fat is dominated by the *Prevotella*.

In studies, when vegetarians were put on an animal diet, and the meat eaters went vegetarian, their microbiomes switched after just twenty-four hours. Researchers at Monash University in Melbourne, Australia, discovered general patterns of gut bacteria called enterotypes, which appear to be influenced by both genetics and the diet you've been eating for most of your life. So far, they have identified three enterotypes: *Bacteroides* dominant, *Prevotella* dominant, and *Ruminococcus* dominant, and they don't seem to be influenced by body mass index, age, gender, or geographical location. It appears that you develop an enterotype over the long term. This suggests that there might be a limited number of gut microbe patterns and, similar to having a body type, you might have a specific "default" enterotype. It is still unknown if there is a connection between any given enterotype and disease, but this is the next step in this area of research.[11]

The message here is that changing your gut flora is a stubborn process, and since that is what we are trying to do as part of the Arthritis Protocol, it is a reminder that this will take time. Think of your enterotype as the underlying terrain—the soil in your gut. It may take years to shift your enterotype or to create a permanent change in your gut bacteria. Step 1, the Two-Week Jump-Start Leaky Gut Diet for Arthritis, gives you a kick start. But step 3, the Finish-What-You-Started Six-Month Program, moves you into the lifelong dietary changes you will need to make to permanently improve your gut bacteria so that the new pattern becomes your default.

Others studies have found that people within families share the same pattern of bacteria, supporting the idea that enterotypes remain stable as part of the gut foundation; while the flora might change with diet or other factors in the short run, it always tries to return to its original enterotype.[12] This is why adopting an anti-inflammatory, gut-healthy diet needs to be a permanent change. In other words, quick fixes such as short-term special diets or weight loss programs never work.

A lot of communication takes place between your gut bacteria and the rest of your body. Your immune system recognizes bacterial surface molecules and DNA, so that it knows these are friendly flora. The cross communication enables the bacteria and your cells to recognize one another. This is very important for maintaining balance in both the gut and the immune system. The bacteria also communicate by making molecules called metabolites; these are end products of diet-dependent bacterial metabolism, which is why diet affects your health in such a big way. The bacteria convert nutrients into these metabolites, which then exert a direct effect on the immune system in your gut and on your health via the gut.[13]

For example, a very important group of metabolites made by your good flora, called short-chain fatty acids (SCFA), are estimated to provide 10 percent of the energy supply in humans. The process goes like this: indigestible carbohydrates (such as the almost woody, fibrous cellulose in vegetables like celery) that escape digestion in the small intestine make their way to the colon. There, bacteria called Firmicutes, Bacteroidetes, and *Bifidobacterium* make short-chain fatty acids—specifically the three most important ones: butyrate, the primary energy source for colonic epithelial cells, as well as propionate and acetate.

The amounts and types of short-chain fatty acids are determined by the kinds of bacteria in the gut and the food you eat. For example, in the uppermost part of the colon, the bacteria ferment the carbs in the diet and maybe SCFA's. But if carbs are depleted—which can happen by the time the semi-solid waste matter reaches the end of the colon, to be excreted—the bacteria metabolize protein instead and make potentially harmful compounds such as ammonia. This can build up and cause symptoms like fatigue, nausea, headache, and muscle weakness. Some of these compounds may also be involved in colon cancer or inflammatory bowel disease. A diet high in animal protein and processed flour products and low in produce (which is the standard American diet) would not provide enough fiber to feed the bacteria sufficiently to support your gut health and overall wellness. The large amount of protein could also be processed into toxic levels of ammonia.

High levels of short-chain fatty acids also inhibit *Escherichia coli* (*E. coli*) and *Salmonella* and create a favorable environment in the colon for bacterial growth and healthy immune function. Butyrate and propionate are key players in regulating intestinal permeability and can help fill the holes in a leaky gut by repairing the tight junctions and stimulating production of a compound that strengthens the barrier. Butyrate can also help reduce inflammation by directly affecting the gut lining and by triggering an increase in T regulator cells, which help reduce inflammation.[14]

T regulator cells are a subgroup of white blood cells known as T cells, the body's foot soldiers against infection. They are tasked with regulating the various populations of T cells and preventing your immune system from attacking your own tissues, a situation that leads to autoimmune disease. As a result, they need to help create and maintain something called tolerance, which is when your body can decipher what is foreign and what isn't. And in this role, they can help turn off autoimmune responses. I dedicated a whole section of my last book to explaining the role and importance of T regulator cells. For more details on this subject, I refer you to that book. Here, I want to share the importance of these T regulator cells in modulating all the activity of the immune system, in their role in autoimmunity, and in the importance of the gut flora in helping them develop and work properly in an ongoing way. *You will not have well-functioning T regulators unless your gut bacteria and intestinal barrier are functioning well, too.* Period. This underlying mechanism is extremely important when you have a systemic inflammatory condition such as arthritis and even more so if it is an autoimmune disease such as rheumatoid arthritis.

A study by the Howard Hughes Medical Institute and Ludwig Center at Memorial Sloan Kettering Cancer Center in New York investigated the effect of butyrate on the T regulator cells. Researchers gave oral butyrate to mice, which triggered a significant increase in the T regulator cells released outside of the gut—especially from the spleen (where T cells and other immune cells are stored) and the lymph nodes (where T regulator and other immune cells are made).

The results confirmed another connection and evidence that the gut flora, via its production of butyrate and other short-chain fatty acids, can have a far-reaching influence on the immune system and auto-immunity throughout the body. Interestingly, for the maximum local effect on the colonic epithelial cells and tight junctions, butyrate worked best if given by enema instead of orally. This tells me that it is better to help the bacteria make butyrate in the colon by eating a high-fiber diet rather than taking a butyrate supplement, showing yet again that changing your diet trumps taking a supplement every time![15]

Additional studies have shown that in mice with no gut flora, low short-chain fatty acids are accompanied by impaired development of T regulators. And then when the mice were given butyrate or had their bacteria restored, both situations resulted in restoring the number of T regulators. This again highlights the importance of short-chain fatty acids—especially butyrate—producing bacteria in the gut. And remember, in order to make the short-chain fatty acids, you need both to have these bacteria present in good numbers *and* to feed them properly. A Mediterranean-style diet, which is high in fruit, vegetables, and legumes (the seed from a leguminous plant like peas, beans, and peanuts), and low in meat and saturated fats, has been shown to increase the levels of fecal SCFA.[16]

In addition to making short-chain fatty acids to support the immune system, the intestinal flora makes other compounds, including vitamins. Each species of bacteria appears to colonize a specific niche and has a potential different purpose. Although we are just beginning to understand this, we do know that we have a mutually beneficial relationship. We provide nourishment to the bacteria, and they help us digest and assimilate our food, while also producing vitamins and nutrients that we need. For example, one study found that a specific species of *Bacteroides* help digest lettuce and onions, nutrients that would otherwise be indigestible.[17] In addition, both *Bifidobacteria* and *Lactobacilli* can make folate (also known as vitamin B_9). Vitamins are also needed for the health of the gut immune system. A deficiency of vitamin A and its activated form, retinoic acid, cause a susceptibility to infections and increased mortality because of impaired immunity in the intestinal mucosa. Retinoic acid helps to improve microbiota diversity and to increase T regulators. Vitamins D, B$_{12}$, and folate also support T regulator cells in the gut.[18]

The beneficial bacteria in your gut have several other very important immune functions. They provide direct antibacterial action against disease-causing pathogens and stimulate epithelial and immune cells to increase production of the antibody immunoglobulin A (IgA), which helps protect against pathogens, too. IgA is the main type of antibody in the gut, mouth, and lungs. It is considered a major player in the gut immune system and binds to viruses and bacteria to prevent or inhibit their attachment and invasion into the body. IgA also reduces inflammation in the intestinal mucosa, and, in all these ways, helps prevent a leaky gut. Gut bacteria are key players in helping the B lymphocyte plasma cells that make IgA mature and function properly. Peyer's patches are areas in the gut where plasma cells live and where most of IgA is manufactured, although it is also made throughout the gut lining. In mice that don't have any IgA, their gut bacteria expands a hundredfold in all areas of the small intestine! This highlights the role of IgA in keeping your good flora in check, because too much of a good thing can be harmful. In fact, the researchers found that this bacterial overgrowth led to overactivation of both the gut and whole body immune systems. When IgA-producing cells were reintroduced, the overgrowth normalized, and the authors concluded that increasing gut IgA could be a novel way to treat gut dysbiosis.[19] Because probiotics have been shown to increase IgA, it may be one of the ways that probiotics help treat dysbiosis.

How do your immune cells recognize your gut bacteria as friend or foe? It appears that immune cells sample the contents of the gut all the time, and this is how they learn to ignore the good bacteria, a situation called tolerance. We have long known that there are patterns on the surface of the bacteria that are recognized as foreign or familiar by our immune system, but it turns out that bacterial DNA can also directly increase or decrease T regulators and suppress our inflammatory responses. This suggests that the potential for dysbiosis to cause disease may be due to an increase in immunostimulatory DNA or immunosuppressive DNA from gut flora, and this can be the final straw that tips the balance in the gut toward inflammation. Researchers from the National Institutes of Health (NIH) in Bethesda, Maryland, found that the good bacterial DNA from *Lactobacillus* species, *Bacteroides fragilis*, and a good species of *Clostridium* could increase T regulator cells, and that the DNA from *Lactobacillus paracasei* was able to protect the mice from parasitic infection.[20]

Gut Bacteria and Arthritis

Now that you understand the anatomy of your digestive system and importance of a strong intestinal barrier and gut bacteria, let's talk about the gut-arthritis connection. First, we'll discuss dysbiosis, a condition in which the gut bacteria don't have enough of the robust and healthy bacteria they need and have an overgrowth of harmful bacteria, yeast, or parasites. Dysbiosis is the missing link to making the connection between what can go wrong in the gut and the outcome of what becomes arthritis.

You can have dysbiosis without having any digestive symptoms. This is the case with many people with arthritis and autoimmune disease. This is why anybody who has one of these conditions should treat dysbiosis even without symptoms or any tests (such as a stool test) to confirm the diagnosis. Dysbiosis can be caused by stress, antibiotics, antacids, proton pump inhibitors, gut infections (traveler's diarrhea, for example), and diet. The only way to really cure arthritis at the root cause is to treat the dysbiosis and bring your gut bacteria to a state of balance and health, because dysbiosis is a source of ongoing inflammation throughout the body.[21]

Extensive research has revealed a link between RA and dysbiosis. Not only does this cause gut inflammation, but dysbiosis also leads to a damaged intestinal lining, causing a leaky gut, which then allows components of intestinal bacteria to travel through the bloodstream to other parts of the body. Dysbiosis represents an altered state of gut bacteria, and all the good activities that should be helping your gut barrier stay strong and your immune system stay balanced are just not happening like they should. Eventually this leads to inflammation throughout the body, including the joints, something that has been confirmed by studies where cell wall components of gut bacteria were actually found in joint synovial fluid.[22] These components are believed to trigger oxidative stress and more inflammation, causing pain, swelling, and ultimately joint damage.

It is clear that dysbiosis is an important trigger for inflammatory arthritis. But there are many different types of dysbiosis, which researchers are trying to identify in order to develop and create targeted treatments. Is it a general imbalance in the flora, with many different species that are either overabundant, too low, or in short supply? Or are there specific patterns of the different species that correspond to different types of arthritis? Or could there be one particular bacteria or a few specific bacteria that could be the culprits in triggering RA? Back in 1987, the earliest study I could find on this topic, researchers at the University of Leeds in the United Kingdom found that people with rheumatoid arthritis had much higher levels of *Clostridium perfringens* than people without RA, as well as significantly higher counts than those with inactive disease. Interestingly, this was before we had the ability to really examine gut microbes![23] But it took a while for the focus on the gut bacteria as the origin of immune and inflammatory diseases to catch on, and in the past decade, there have been many more studies identifying different kinds of bacteria as possible culprits.

In chapter 1, "Rheumatoid Arthritis," we discussed *P. mirabilis*, a bacteria living in the gut that appears to have the ability to initiate the autoimmune events associated with RA.[24] Recent studies have also identified a gut bacteria called *Prevotella copri* as a possible trigger for RA. Keep in mind that having too much of this *Prevotella* in your gut doesn't mean you will get rheumatoid arthritis. I often see patients with stool test results high in *Prevotella*, yet they don't have RA. This could be because they don't have the genes that make them susceptible to getting it.

Researchers from Osaka University in Japan also discovered that certain RA patients had gut microbes dominated by this bacteria strain, which can trigger immune cells to cause joint inflammation. This study demonstrates clearly that bacteria in the gut can cause reactions in immune cells outside the intestines, and this process was a trigger for developing RA. The findings support current efforts to find ways to treat the gut microbiota as an approach to treating rheumatoid arthritis. One technique being studied is called fecal microbiota transplantation (FMT), which is currently being used to treat people with an infection called *Clostridium difficile*. While the authors don't suggest using fecal transplant in RA patients, they underscore the idea of treating dysbiosis as a way of treating RA. I will tell you more about fecal transplant in chapter 6 on treatment. You can see how this and the other research I am sharing in this book provide medical proof that healing the gut is the right approach for treating arthritis and show you why the gut is the foundation of the Arthritis Protocol.[25]

When researchers at the Chinese Academy of Medical Sciences and Peking Union Medical College in Beijing compared the gut and oral bacteria of symptomatic RA sufferers with those of a healthy group, they discovered a specific pattern of gut and oral dysbiosis in the RA group. They found high levels of *Lactobacillus salivarius*, *Atopobium* spp., and *Cryptobacterium curtum* in saliva and dental samples from the RA group, while the healthy group had higher amounts of different bacteria—specifically *Neisseria* spp. and *Rothia aeria*. The patterns of bacteria in the gut, too, were different for the two groups.

Interestingly, the authors also evaluated the gut bacteria of patients before and after taking methotrexate, a conventional RA medication, and found that it partially restored the gut bacteria. What's more, these changes predicted better results (in RA symptoms) from the treatment. This brings up the interesting possibility that the medication might be exerting its effect by improving the gut bacteria. The authors concluded that RA represents a state of chronic inflammation that might be provoked or aggravated by the overgrowth of bad bacteria or a lack of good bacteria in both the mouth and the gut.[26] Other medications might also work, not only by suppressing the immune system and inflammation but by positively altering the gut bacteria. Sulfasalazine (Azulfidine), a combination of aspirin and sulfa antibiotic, and the antimalarial hydroxychloroquine (Plaquenil) are both used as anti-inflammatory medications, and it seems very likely that alterations in the gut bacteria play a part in their positive results.

A review study by researchers at Christian Medical College in Tamil Nadu, India, found that RA patients had high levels of *Clostridium perfringens* when compared with the control group in four different studies and that treatment with sulfasalazine decreased counts in two of these studies. It certainly seems that changes in the gut flora are a part of the effect of these medications.[27] In psoriatic arthritis, just like in rheumatoid arthritis, having dysbiosis, a damaged intestinal lining, and/or leaky gut may be to blame. More and more studies confirm these connections, and researchers are suggesting approaches such as antibiotic treatment, probiotic and prebiotic delivery, and even fecal transplant to treat systemic inflammation by manipulating the microbiota.[28] I hope you are now beginning to see that gut bacteria research has the potential to revolutionize research, diagnosis, and treatment of all inflammatory arthritis conditions.

Regarding ankylosing spondylitis, multiple studies have found dysbiosis with alterations in the amounts of different bacteria that are considered part of the normal flora. Specifically, researchers saw an increase of Lachnospiraceae, Prevotellaceae, and *Ruminococcus* in AS patients, and a decrease of *Streptococcus* and *Actinomyces*. In another study, there was an increase in *Bacteroides*.[29] Again, until researchers can conclusively connect different patterns of dysbiosis with different diseases, my point isn't to focus on the exact strains of bacteria that were out of balance but to demonstrate that dysbiosis is a common feature in those with inflammatory arthritis and appears to trigger a whole cascade of inflammation that ends up in the joints. The functional medicine approach to treating dysbiosis is to use broad-spectrum herbs, so it isn't necessary to know exactly which bacteria need to be eliminated. Now that it's become clear that dysbiosis and the resulting leaky gut can cause arthritis, we can treat the root cause (the gut) and not just what's on the surface (arthritis symptoms).

Studies of people with inflammatory bowel disease (IBD) provide more evidence connecting the gut and arthritis. IBD, in which chronic inflammation affects all or part of the digestive tract, includes Crohn's disease, which afflicts the small intestine, and ulcerative colitis, which takes hold in the large intestine, or colon. Up to 10 percent of people with IBD develop ankylosing spondylitis, and it is more common in people with AS and rheumatoid arthritis than in the general population and in those with other autoimmune diseases, such as lupus and Sjögren's syndrome. Clearly, among all autoimmune diseases, the gut connection is strongest in those with autoimmune inflammatory arthritis.[30]

One final word about dysbiosis. Small intestinal bacterial overgrowth (SIBO) is a specific type of dysbiosis that has gotten a lot of attention in the past few years because more and more people have it. SIBO usually affects the upper part of the small intestine, and its hallmark is symptoms such as a gurgling sensation in the abdomen, gas, and bloating within ninety minutes of having eaten. Often the overgrowth involves good bacteria that have ended up in the wrong place. Nevertheless, this interferes with normal functioning of the small bowel, causing malabsorption of fat and nutrients and leading to vitamin deficiencies, like B vitamins and antioxidants, which can lead to an increased risk of fatigue and oxidative stress. It is also likely that it can cause a leaky gut, because the small intestine has a very thin protective mucous layer, making it likely that the overgrown bacteria come into contact with the epithelial cell surface, thus triggering increased intestinal permeability. This condition was identified relatively recently, so we don't know if it is associated with arthritis. Still, when someone has SIBO, including my patients with arthritis,

I treat it until it is resolved, following the same herbal program that I use to treat dysbiosis. However, people with SIBO often need multiple courses of treatment.

Lastly, emerging research is beginning to link the gut bacteria to osteoarthritis. As explained in chapter 3, "Osteoarthritis," OA is considered a metabolic disease that is associated with having excess body fat, obesity, diabetes, and metabolic syndrome. All of this represents a disordered state of glucose and fat metabolism in the body, and the process appears to cause joint inflammation and erosion. Recent research has linked obesity to changes in the gut bacteria. For example, scientists at Canada's University of Calgary studied the role that gut microbiota might play in initiating and driving the inflammation of osteoarthritis. They found that rats who were fed a diet high in fat and table sugar became obese and developed a much different gut flora pattern than that of nonobese rats who'd been put on a diet lower in fat and sugar. The obese animals had higher body fat, lower levels of *Lactobacillus* species, and higher scores for OA. Conversely, the higher the level of *Lactobacillus* species, the lower the scores not only for osteoarthritis but also for inflammatory markers in the blood and synovial fluid, and for leptin, the inflammatory molecule released by fat cells.

Another species of bacteria that was identified, *Methanobrevibacter*, seemed to have the opposite effect: high levels were associated with inflammation and high arthritis scores. The researchers also found that obese rats had high levels of pieces of the cell walls of gut bacteria in their blood (sometimes called serum lipopolysaccharide (LPS), and this was a good marker for the presence of leaky gut.[31] This study shows that dysbiosis and leaky gut are also likely to be involved in some way with the onset and progression of OA. Given that we know leaky gut triggers systemic inflammation, it would be important to include gut repair in people with osteoarthritis, too.

Now, let's come back to how I treated June. When I used my medical detective skills to dive into her past and present, I found out that she had been healthy throughout her childhood in Pittsburgh, without any digestive or immune issues. In her early twenties, while living in Japan and Hawaii, June developed ulcerative colitis with diarrhea, cramps, and weight loss, but then she moved to Guyana at the age of twenty-seven, and her symptoms resolved while she lived there. Once she got married, her husband's job with the United Nations took them to various countries around the world for four or five years at a time. In her early thirties, she moved to New York and still felt well, but, at thirty-seven, she and her family moved to Yemen. During her four years there, June developed a bad case of diarrhea, which was caused by a parasite called an amoeba. Their next destination? Nepal, where she struggled with the parasitic infection giardia on and off for five years, and her four children were treated for worms multiple times. When she was forty-seven, her family moved to Connecticut, where they lived for the next fifteen years. There she saw a parasite special-ist who found and treated her for infections (she couldn't remember which ones), and, as a result, she had no digestive issues. Once her husband retired when she was sixty-two, they moved to Malaysia, where she taught English as a second language for four years. Three years ago, she moved back to Connecticut with her family.

But it wasn't just her surroundings that changed dramatically—so did June's diet. She started drinking alcohol, mostly wine, and went from consuming an Asian diet consisting of little dairy and lots of soy, fish, rice, and vegetables to eating more dairy and processed foods when she moved back to the States. The latter is what we call the standard American diet, and it's not a healthy one. Dairy, gluten, and alcohol can increase inflammation in the body, and gluten and alcohol can cause a leaky gut. (I will talk more about this in chapter 7, "Food and Fire.")

At first, she was happy in her new teaching job back in the United States, but the school she worked in had no heat, her hands began to hurt, and her fingers turned blue in the winter. This was the first sign that something was wrong. She was diagnosed with Raynaud's disease, an autoimmune condition in which the smaller arteries that deliver oxygen-rich blood to the skin constrict in the cold. This also limits oxygen flow to the joints, which may have contributed to the onset of her arthritis.[32]

Then June broke her toe while exercising, and instead of healing, it became arthritic. Shortly after this, she developed pain and swelling in her hands that was not related to the cold, and then in her shoulder and knee. She went to the rheumatologist, was diagnosed with RA, and thus began her journey into medication. When strong prescription drugs such as methotrexate and hydroxychloroquine (Plaquenil) didn't work, and caused side effects such as hard-to-heal, painful canker sores and brittle hair and nails, she tried the corticosteroid prednisone. This was the only thing that helped her function, but I use the word "function" loosely, because as I shared earlier, she couldn't open jars, use scissors, or get dressed without her husband's help! Although her symptoms *appeared* to have nothing to do with her digestive system, June's issues—and those of most rheumatoid arthritis sufferers—began in her gut. Even without the test results that later revealed severe dysbiosis, I knew this was likely the foundational cause of her RA. Then the triggers from an inflammatory diet, stress, physical trauma in her fingers from the Raynaud's, and the broken toe conspired to put her over the top and trigger her arthritis symptoms. The bottom line? First, we needed to focus on June's gut health.

To treat the dysbiosis, we used herbs (see the sidebar for my favorite herbs, on page 105) which is the main treatment approach that is used in the Arthritis Protocol. To treat her leaky gut, June took glutamine powder, an amino acid that nourishes the cells that line the intestines and repairs the lining. She also had *Candida*, which, as I mentioned previously, is a kind of yeast that can cause an infection in the gut and trigger inflammation and leaky gut too. For this, we used a prescription antifungal medication called nystatin, which goes by several brand names, including Mycostatin. June also took a probiotic at night. In the Arthritis Protocol, we always begin with food because it has the power to really help relieve symptoms quickly. As a result, June started with the Leaky Gut Diet for Arthritis, which is an elimination diet to determine if any common foods—such as dairy, eggs, gluten, corn, and soy—were triggering her symptoms. She also avoided nightshade vegetables, which include tomatoes, pota-toes, eggplant, and peppers, because these are believed to contain compounds that trigger inflammation and arthritis symptoms. When June stuck to the diet, her symptoms improved. But when she was stressed at her job and couldn't follow the dietary plan completely, they got worse.

After thirteen months, she felt great. "I could live this way for the rest of my life," she told me. Our primary goal at that point was con-tinuing to treat her gut until the dysbiosis was gone based on the stool test, which would help to prevent another flare-up (also called a relapse), and to help her taper off medication. Healing the gut often requires several rounds of treatment, and for her bacterial and yeast dysbiosis to finally be cured *based on her stool test*, it took June five separate one- to two-month treatments of gut herbs over a twenty-one-month period. (See the sidebar on page 105 for the details.) But at long last, we achieved all these goals. I believe that in addition to the gut treatment, the dietary changes really made a difference, too. Even though she went off the plan many times, June was still eating a lot less dairy, gluten, and sugar than before.

It's very exciting for me and my functional medicine colleagues to see research finally catching up with what we have been doing. For almost two decades, my main approach to treating people with inflammatory conditions has been to focus on repairing gut flora and treating leaky gut. My patient Sherry, whom you met in chapter 1, is another example.

As a child, Sherry had frequent stomachaches and took a variety of antibiotics for strep throat, a common bacterial infection in children. At thirteen, she contracted a bad case of traveler's diarrhea that took months to go away, and had cramps and diarrhea on and off through-out college and into her twenties. It also seemed that every time she went on vacation, she would experience digestive issues. In her thir-ties, the mother of two from New York City constantly felt exhausted and began having pain in her toes and feet. These symptoms came on slowly but steadily. Eventually, at the age of forty, Sherry was diagnosed with rheumatoid arthritis. Just like June, she clearly had a history of gut problems. After listening to her story, it was clear to me that dysbiosis in her gut from an overgrowth of harmful bacteria, possibly parasites and yeast, was the likely trigger for her disease. With both women, like so many of my patients, repairing their gut flora was the primary strategy for healing their joints and inflammation.

The Oral Microbiome

Although my patients come to me to teach them how to improve their health, I often learn a lot from them. One in particular is Debbie, a fifty-two-year-old woman with rheumatoid arthritis. She came to see me with joint pain in her left wrist, both ankles, neck, and right shoulder, and hand stiffness that had been bothering her for seven years. These symptoms began after she'd had six silver mercury amalgam fillings removed from her mouth. She also had severe periodontal disease and went regularly to a specialist to have her gums treated. The Plaquenil that Debbie tried not only didn't stop the pain but actually made matters worse: she kept getting sick a lot and complained of fatigue, so she stopped taking it. Because she had no history of gut issues and no digestive symptoms, I thought her RA might have been triggered by mercury released when her dentist removed the fillings. As I describe in great detail in my first book, *The Immune System Recovery Plan*, mercury is a heavy metal that can trigger autoimmunity and is associated with autoimmune diseases, including Hashimoto's thyroiditis. While mercury hasn't been well studied as a cause of RA, it is a known trigger for autoimmunity, so I felt this was a possibility. Debbie agreed, because the arthritis came on almost immediately after her intense amount of dental work. It turns out that we were both wrong. While I do believe her RA was related to her dental work, I realized that it was not specifically due to the release of mercury. Instead, the cause was her oral microbiome and worsening periodontal issues.

However, I didn't realize this at first. After testing revealed that Debbie had high mercury levels, her treatment focused on a liver detox program for the next eight months to get the metals out. This consisted of taking supplements and herbs that provide nutrients to help the liver remove mercury and other toxins. (For more information on this, read *The Immune System Recovery Plan*, "Step 4: Supporting Your Liver.") She also began the basic anti-inflammatory program that I use in the Arthritis Protocol, with high doses of omega oils, vitamin D, and probiotics. Her pain began to improve, but she was only partly better by the end of the eight months. While blood tests showed improvement in some of her inflammatory markers, her ACPA (anti-citrullinated peptide antibody) blood test stubbornly remained greater than 250 units. (Normal is less than 18 units.) This is very high (a "strong positive" is a result greater than 60 units), so I did some research. I discovered that there is an association between periodontal disease and bacterial imbalance in the oral microbiome (microorganisms found in the mouth) in people with rheumatoid arthritis, and these patients tend to have high ACPA levels. A bacterium called *Porphyromonas gingivalis*, which has been found in higher levels in RA patients than those without the disease, produces enzymes that can damage tissue in the body, leading to an autoimmune response. (Smoking cigarettes is believed to boost these enzymes, which explains why smoking is the number one risk factor for RA.)[33] Support for this hypothesis came from the University of Bergen, in Norway, where researchers found the DNA of oral bacteria in the synovial fluid of patients with rheumatoid arthritis or psoriatic arthritis, but not in healthy study participants.[34]

It became clear to me that the release of bacteria from Debbie's gums during her dental procedures triggered her RA. And even though she didn't have a history of gut issues or current symptoms, swallowing all those bad bacteria was likely filling her gut with harmful microbes, too. Given the emerging science and understanding about the importance of the oral microbiome and periodontal disease in rheumatoid arthritis, I needed to treat her mouth *and* her gut. When I did, she finally felt a big improvement in her joint pain. Since then, all my patients with periodontal disease or dental/gum issues, and especially those with a positive ACPA blood test, go on an oral microbiome treatment program as part of their Arthritis Protocol. I will show you how to do this in our comprehensive treatment program.

CHAPTER 6

How to Heal the Gut

There is no doubt that the gut bacteria are involved in the onset and perpetuation of inflammation and pain in arthritis. Because this evidence is so strong and compelling, researchers have taken it to the next step by asking, "Does treating the gut also treat arthritis?" The studies are fascinating and satisfying for me because my functional medicine colleagues and I have been working to heal the gut bacteria for decades—and many other practitioners of natural medicine, such as herbalists and naturopaths, were doing so even before us. I am extremely gratified to see that healing the gut to treat arthritis and inflammation has become a topic in the medical literature and is validated by science. However, the studies to date are limited, in my opinion, because they don't approach healing the gut in a comprehensive way and certainly not as effectively as my fellow practitioners and I do. Even so, the results prove to me that following the Arthritis Protocol is even more effective than what this research highlights.

This chapter focusing on gut treatment is divided into three sections. First, we will review the studies using probiotics to alter the gut bacteria and environment as a way to treat arthritis. We will also look at additional studies on the impact of probiotics on the gut, in general, as a way to explore the different strains and to share what I think are the best probiotic supplements. Next, we will review how to treat dysbiosis and leaky gut with herbs and supplements other than probiotics, which is what you will do in the Arthritis Protocol. Finally, we will return to my patients' stories and the exact programs they followed. Your diet and stress management (or lack thereof) are also key players in healing your gut and arthritis, so each has its own chapter. In chapter 7, "Food and Fire," we'll review the many studies that reveal a link between diet and arthritis, and in chapter 8, "Traumatic Stress: Fueling the Fire," I'll explain the relationship between trauma, stress, and arthritis.

Before we begin, I want to point out that to successfully treat dysbiosis, you must remove the original reason that you got this condition in the first place. In other words, if you are taking antibiotics, antacids, or a proton pump inhibitor such as omeprazole (brand name, Prevacid) or lansoprazole (Prilosec) regularly, you need to stop as soon as possible. Reflux is often caused by a combination of dysbiosis and food triggers, which is why, after you start the step 1 Two-Week Jump-Start Leaky Gut Diet for Arthritis, followed by step 2, the Two-Month Intensive Gut Repair, which treats the dysbiosis, you should be able to stop these medications within a few weeks without your reflux recurring.

Treating Arthritis with Probiotics

The term "dysbiosis" was introduced more than a century ago by the Russian biologist and Nobel Prize laureate Elie Metchnikoff, who coined it to describe a disruption of the normal balance of the bacteria in the gut. Metchnikoff, referred to as the father of natural immunity, then proposed using yogurt with active bacterial cultures to improve both the gut and human health.[1]

Probiotics are living bacteria normally found in the human digestive tract that are ingested to improve the quality and quantity of the gut's beneficial bacteria. They can be ingested as part of the diet, in foods like yogurt, or taken in supplement form for therapeutic purposes. The goal is to shift the population of gut bacteria toward one that is more healing and low inflammatory. Probiotics can improve leaky gut, reduce intestinal permeability, and help increase the production of the short-chain fatty acid butyrate. In addition, taking probiotics also reduces proinflammatory bacteria such as *Escherichia coli*, *Enterobacter aerogenes*, *Klebsiella pneumoniae*, *Streptococcus viridans*, *Bacteroides fragilis*, *Bacteroides uniformis*, and *Clostridium ramosum*. When these and other potentially harmful bacteria are present in high amounts, they trigger dysbiosis.[2] Probiotic supplements are one way that researchers have treated the dysbiosis of inflammatory arthritis, and it certainly seems like a good place to start. However, not all probiotics are the same because many different strains of bacteria can be used. Currently, probiotic research is determining which strains are most important for which conditions. Various strains can either turn up or turn down your immune system function. *Generally speaking, when it comes to arthritis, probiotics are thought to improve all the functions of the good flora that we reviewed, including helping T regulator immune cells work better and live longer, turning off inflammation, and repairing the gut lining and tight junctions.* Because probiotics help treat a leaky gut, it follows that they would also treat systemic inflammation and arthritis.

Researchers at Tabriz University of Medical Science in Iran reviewed all the studies looking at the use of probiotics to treat rheumatoid arthritis. Using different probiotic strains, four randomized double-blind, placebo-controlled trials showed that treatment with *Lactobacillus rhamnosus GG*, *Lactobacillus rhamnosus GR-1*, and *Lactobacillus reuteri RC-14* improved patients' well-being but didn't change pain scores or inflammatory markers. One month of *Bacillus coagulans* improved pain and patient global assessment scores and reduced inflammatory markers. Treatment with *Lactobacillus casei* for eight weeks improved pain scores and reduced inflammatory markers and cytokine levels. These studies clearly show that using probiotics for only a short period of time had a recognizable effect on both RA symptoms and disease markers, depending on which strains were used.[3]

Early studies on *Lactobacillus casei* appeared so promising that numerous researchers have continued to look at it. According to one such study, treatment of rheumatoid arthritis with *L. casei* significantly lowered pro-inflammatory cells, increased the anti-inflammatory cytokine interleukin-10 (IL-10), and significantly decreased pain scores.[4] In another study, it reduced measures of inflammation and the number of tender and swollen joints. There were also improvements in inflammation markers and improved DAS28, the disease activity scoring system for symptoms that you learned about in chapter 1. While studies have not looked at dosing, this study used one daily capsule of 100 million CFU for eight weeks—a low dose by current standards—which highlights that more is not necessarily better.[5] CFU is an abbreviation for "colony-forming units" and is used to quantify how many bacteria in probiotics are capable of dividing and forming colonies.

Researchers at the University of Western Ontario studied rheumatoid arthritis and two probiotic strains, *Lactobacillus rhamnosus* and *Lactobacillus reuteri*, in this three-month double-blind, placebo-controlled study. They had fifteen subjects in the probiotic group and fifteen in the control group. All participants had four tender and swollen joints, hadn't had any recent changes in medication, and had not taken steroids for at least one month prior to and during the study. When researchers looked at joint symptoms, blood levels of inflammation markers called serum cytokines, and a health assessment questionnaire having to do with activities of daily life, they found improvement in the written self-assessments, suggesting a possible positive effect on their quality of life and ability to function.[6]

In addition to the arthritis studies recruiting men and women, there have been many rat studies as well. In animals, it is easier to learn the probiotics' action, too. Researchers at Tel Aviv University in Israel studied the effect of probiotics on rats that are bred specifically for their genetic predisposition to inflammatory arthritis, called Lewis rats. Results revealed that the anti-inflammatory effects of *Lactobacillus GG* (a specific strain also called *Lactobacillus rhamnosus GG*) on arthritis did not depend on whether the bacteria were alive or killed by heat. This is fascinating because we are always very concerned about probiotics being refrigerated in order to keep the cultures alive, and this study suggests that—at least for the anti-inflammatory effects—living bacteria might not be necessary. The researchers believe that it must be parts of the cell wall or some other part of the bacteria that have the effect on the immune system. They also found that the probiotic was more effective in reducing arthritis inflammation when it was given to the rats in cultured dairy such as yogurt, suggesting that the bacteria might be secreting something that lives in the food, and this adds to the effect. Of course, this supports my view that using food as medicine is the best way to stay in balance for both prevention and maintenance and as part of the repair and healing process, which we will talk more about in the next chapter, "Food and Fire."

There were other interesting findings, such as that the probiotic effect on the immune system gets stronger the longer you take the food or supplement and that this also improves the healthy development of your lymphocytes (one of several different types of white blood cells) in the gut and reduces their reactions to food antigens. They also reinforced what other studies have shown: that probiotics help regulate the release of messenger molecules called cytokines, which can be either anti-inflammatory or pro-inflammatory. And because probiotics help regulate this balance, they are very good for treating allergies.[7]

When researchers from the Barkatullah University in Bhopal, Madhya Pradesh, India, gave *Lactobacillus casei* to female rats, they found that it protected them against arthritis symptoms, while in rats already affected with arthritis, it reduced their footpad swelling and redness and improved their mobility. In this study, they measured anti- and pro-inflammatory cytokines and found that *L. casei* significantly decreased secretion of the pro-inflammatory cytokines TNF-alpha and interleukin-6, and appeared to inhibit the COX-2 pathway and activation of nuclear factor kappa B (NFkB). Both of these are potent inflammatory messengers in the body that are known to be associated with rheumatoid arthritis and osteoarthritis, and are the driving forces behind the damage to cartilage and bone.[8] When the same group of researchers looked at the effect of *Lactobacillus acidophilus* in these animals, they found that giving *L. acidophilus* protected against damage to the joints, which is believed to result from systemic inflammation. TNF-alpha seems to be the main villain behind this process, and *L. acidophilus* was able to block it and suppress inflammation. IL-6 is another cytokine involved in joint destruction, and *L. acidophilus* inhibited this one, too.[9]

Researchers from Gwangju Institute of Science and Technology, in South Korea, found that rats with osteoarthritis who were given oral *Lactobacillus casei* had reduced levels of inflammation and cartilage breakdown, which supports the role of using probiotics and/or repairing gut flora as part of OA treatment.[10] These encouraging studies are a first baby step toward the wider acceptance of improving the gut bacteria as a central strategy for treating arthritis of all kinds. The next question is "What do we know about the different probiotic strains and which are the best choices?"

Probiotics and Gut Health

Probiotics have been studied for other gut-related health conditions, including ulcerative colitis, Crohn's disease, small intestinal bacterial overgrowth, and leaky gut. Researchers at Ireland's University College at Cork studied a strain of *Lactobacillus salivarius* isolated from the human intestinal tract and found that it is able to bind to the intestinal epithelial cells and trigger the release of several anti-inflammatory compounds and mucin, the main protein in the mucus that lines the intestines. This supports the idea that gut bacteria influence both your immune system and your intestinal lining.[11] Probiotics that have been studied specifically for their ability to heal and protect the tight junctions and treat leaky gut include *Escherichia coli* Nissle strain, which increased TJ integrity. *Bifidobacterium infantis*, a component of the popular probiotic VSL3, increases occludin, an important protein that fixes damaged tight junctions and thus improves intestinal permeability. A human study on *Lactobacillus plantarum* showed that it triggered an increase in tight junctions.

Other lactobacilli appear to have protective effects on the barrier, including *salivarius, rhamnosus GG,* and *casei.* Probiotics seem to help prevent damage and repair a leaky gut by preventing adhesion of bad bacteria to the intestinal lining, which is protective because these potentially harmful bacteria secrete enzymes that dissolve the tight junctions. They produce inflammation, too, which also degrades the tight junctions. This is why treating dysbiosis is so important.[12]

Other strains have been found to be effective, including a mixture of *Streptococcus thermophilus* and *Lactobacillus acidophilus,* which protected the intestinal barrier against colitis in one experiment. Leaky gut was also improved by the probiotic *Escherichia coli* Nissle 191.[13] Another study showed that *Lactobacillus rhamnosus GG* supplementation improved the mucosal barrier function in the intestine of weaned piglets by protecting the cells and supporting the intestinal microbiota.[14] After reviewing all available studies on the use of probiotics to improve barrier function, researchers from the Fujian Medical University in China found that probiotics can strengthen tight-junction proteins in epithelial cells, increase mucin, and enhance the function of the intestinal EC barrier. They concluded that probiotics should be given preventatively and postoperatively after colon surgery.[15]

The bottom line? The strains researched in arthritis with the most evidence for an anti-inflammatory effect are lactobacilli: *casei, acidophilus, reuteri, rhamnosus GG,* and *salivarius.* There is also good evidence for *Bifidobacterium bifidum. Bifidobacterium infantis, Escherichia coli* Nissle, and *Lactobacillus plantarum* were found to improve tight junctions and heal leaky gut, even if they weren't studied for their effects specifically on arthritis. These data tell me that we are on the right track, that improving the gut microbiota is a good strategy, and that a multistrain formula that includes as many of these as possible, with a priority given to those that have been studied in arthritis patients, is best.

The sidebar below lists my favorite probiotics and the strains included in them. I usually recommend about 20 billion to 30 billion mixed organisms per capsule. Sometimes I use powders for people who prefer this formulation over a pill, or I give a higher dose to someone who has completed a course of antibiotics or who has inflammatory bowel disease. I prefer not to use VSL (the brand name of a very high-potency probiotic that is easily purchased online or in stores) in everyone needing high dosing, because it contains corn starch and maltose, which can cause bloating in people with SIBO or in those who have an intolerance to corn. By far, my preference is the probiotic specialty company Klaire Labs, which I use for my private-label probiotics.

MY FAVORITE PROBIOTICS

Ther-Biotic Complete (twelve strains), from Klaire Labs
- *Lactobacillus rhamnosus*
- *Bifidobacterium bifidum*
- *Lactobacillus acidophilus*
- *Lactobacillus casei*
- *Lactobacillus plantarum*
- *Lactobacillus salivarius*
- *Bifidobacterium longum*
- *Streptococcus thermophilus*
- *Lactobacillus bulgaricus*
- *Lactobacillus paracasei*
- *Bifidobacterium lactis*
- *Bifidobacterium breve*

Ortho Biotic (six strains, nonrefrigerated for travel), from Ortho Molecular Products
- *L. acidophilus*
- *L. paracasei*
- *B. lactis*

- *B. bifidum*
- *L. plantarum*
- *L. rhamnosus*
- *Saccharomyces boulardii*

Probiotic 225 powder, from Ortho Molecular Products
- *L. plantarum*
- *L. acidophilus*
- *B. lactis*
- *L. salivarius*
- *L. casei*
- *B. bifidum*

Treating Dysbiosis

Fecal Transplant

The main focus for our dysbiosis treatment will be using herbal therapies. Before reviewing these, I want to share a treatment on the horizon aiming to improve and repair gut bacteria. It is called fecal microbiota transplantation (FMT), a technique not yet widely available, where stool is taken from a healthy donor and introduced into the patient's body. Currently, researchers are trying to figure out the best way to deliver the fecal material, whether through the mouth or through the rectum. Most preparations are made from whole stool, but researchers are working on encapsulated formulas. It has been used with success to treat the infection *Clostridium difficile*, which up until now has been very difficult to treat. FMT is the first conventional treatment developed specifically to alter the intestinal microbiome, and many scientists have theorized that it could prove useful in patients with other microbiome imbalances, such as inflammatory conditions like rheumatoid arthritis. However, without randomized double-blind placebo-controlled studies, it has not yet been approved in the United States for treating anything other than C. *difficile* and is instead considered an unregulated investigational new drug. Therefore, people wishing to try FMT for a condition other than C. *difficile* would need to travel outside the United States to get it.

Ultimately the goal is to create specific microbe profiles to target specific diseases. Although this is very promising, there are many concerns about long-term safety, and so FMT really isn't ready for widespread use, in my opinion. While there seem to be no short-term adverse effects, there are questions about how to choose the fecal donor and what might be transmitted in a feces sample that we are unable to screen for, such as viruses and other infectious agents. Several of my patients have tried FMT at treatment centers outside the United States, but I have yet to see good results. Nevertheless, to be fair, some of my colleagues have reported success with some of their patients. I do believe this treatment will be very effective someday, but as of this writing, it is still in its infancy.[16]

Herbs

The most effective way to treat dysbiosis is to first remove harmful bacteria or yeast (and sometimes parasites) so that probiotics can be more effective. Think of this as weeding the garden before you plant the flowers. Most studies on using herbal protocols or antibiotics to remove bacteria from the gut have focused on treating small intestinal bacterial overgrowth (which we review on page 85). Many gastroenterologists use rifaximin (brand name, Xifaxan), an oral antibiotic that isn't absorbed into the body but affects the intestines, to treat SIBO, with a cure rate of about 50 percent, according to various studies. It has been shown to be effective against both aerobic and anaerobic bacteria, making it potentially very effective and broad spectrum. The best results have been achieved with doses of 1,200 to 1,600 milligrams daily. The biggest issue is that often many rounds of treatment are needed, and even after the SIBO appears to be gone, it often comes back again.[17] This is very similar to the experiences I have had with many of my patients, including both June and Sherry, who were treated for dysbiosis many times before their gut bacteria finally seemed to be fixed.

But, just like when treating dysbiosis of any kind, it is important to remember that you must address the underlying causes of the SIBO, which mirror those of dysbiosis: diet, stress, low stomach acid, taking antacids, constipation, alcoholism, and, specifically for SIBO, possibly the overuse of high-dose probiotics. Additional causes of SIBO that aren't associated with dysbiosis include systemic diseases that cause nerve damage, impairing the motility of the small intestine and stomach. Motility refers to the movement of the contents through the bowel. Examples include diabetes, damage to the small intestine from surgery or injury, and autoimmune diseases such as scleroderma.[18]

Herbal alternatives to rifaximin have been found to be equally effective, and at the Blum Center for Health, they are our preference because herbs effectively clean out bacteria *and* yeast, while antibiotics target only bacteria and can cause yeast overgrowth as a side effect. Also, over time, it is believed that antibiotic overuse may lead bacteria to develop resistance to these medicines and possibly create an infection with the bacterium *Clostridium difficile*. A study from Johns Hopkins Hospital, in Baltimore, screened a large group of patients in its gastroenterology medical practice and found SIBO in 64 percent. Doctors treated one group of patients with rifaximin and another group with a blend of more than twenty herbs in four different supplements. The cure rate was 46 percent in the herbal treatment group compared with 34 percent for rifaximin. The herbs they used were similar to what we use in the Arthritis Protocol, and included the following:

- Oil of oregano (*Origanum vulgare*) is an herb that has been shown to directly kill or strongly inhibit the growth of intestinal microbes and *Candida*.
- Wormwood (*Artemisia absinthium*) has substantial antimicrobial, antiparasitic, and anti-inflammatory properties.
- Coptis root has growth-inhibitory effects on human bacteria.

- Thyme, which is formulated as both Red thyme essential oil and the whole plant, *Thymus vulgaris*, inhibits the growth of *Escherichia coli*, *Staphylococcus aureus*, and *Candida*.
- Berberine extract and Indian Barberry root extract (*Berberis aristata*) contain berberine, a potent antimicrobial compound.
- Horsetail (*Equisetum arvense*) was shown to possess a broad spectrum of very strong antimicrobial activity against a variety of enteric microorganisms, including *S. aureus*, *E. coli*, *Klebsiella pneumoniae*, *Pseudomonas aeruginosa*, and *Salmonella enteritidis*, and the fungi *Aspergillus niger* and *Candida albicans*.
- *Olea europaea* inhibits the growth of a number of staphylococcal species, including *S. aureus*.[19]

The advantages of herbs go beyond their efficacy. They're generally inexpensive and well tolerated and do not promote yeast. That said, some people experience side effects, so you should carefully monitor anything new that you take and start with the lowest possible dose and work your way up to the full-dose recommendations over several days. While extremely unusual, if you experience nausea, vomiting, or other severe reactions, stop taking them. When your symptoms go away, once you feel better, try a lower dose. If symptoms return, try something completely different from my list: for example, oregano instead of berberine. Never take herbs of any kind if you're pregnant or nursing; don't take berberine if you're also taking an antibiotic, especially azithromycin (Zithromax) or clarithromycin (Biaxin); and check with your doctor before taking herbs if you have liver problems, since many of them are metabolized through this organ. If you're taking multiple medications that induce liver toxicity, such as statins for high cholesterol, ask your doctor to order a liver function blood test before you begin to make sure all is well. It *is* okay to take herbs while on these medications; I'm just overly cautious. Any possible liver irritation is reversible when you stop the herbs, just like what happens when medication causes these same side effects. Most conventional doctors do not understand herbs because they aren't trained or educated in using them, but I still encourage you to tell your doctor what you're doing so that he or she can follow your progress. That said, don't be discouraged if your doctor isn't fully supportive.

Let's explore some of the herbs that have been shown to work in treating dysbiosis and were used in these SIBO studies. Keep in mind, there is a more powerful positive effect on treating dysbiosis when multiple herbs are taken together than if taken separately. This is the way that I use herbs in my practice, and it is the approach used in the successful SIBO studies. Therefore, in general, this is the way that I recommend you use them, too. In this next section, I will review the studies supporting the use of each individual herb and share my favorite blends.

MY FAVORITE HERBAL BLENDS

GI Microb-X, from Designs for Health
- berberine sulfate: 100 milligrams
- barberry (berberine): 50 milligrams
- bearberry extract: 100 milligrams
- tribulus extract: 200 milligrams
- magnesium caprylate: 150 milligrams
- black walnut: 100 milligrams
- artemisinin: 15 milligrams

GI Synergy Packets, from Apex Energetics: proprietary blend, 2,200 milligrams
- wormwood extract
- black walnut extract (hull)
- undecylenic acid
- caprylic acid
- barberry extract (root)
- olive extract (leaf)
- garlic extract (bulb)

- bearberry extract (leaf)
- catclaw extract (bark)
- Pau d'arco extract (bark)
- goldenseal extract (root)
- oregano extract (leaf)
- Oregon grape extract (root)
- Chinese goldthread (*Coptis chinensis*) extract (root)
- yerba mansa (*Anemopsis californica*) extract (leaf)

CandiBactin-BR (good for those allergic to walnut), from Metagenics
- berberine HCL: 400 milligrams
- Coptis (berberine): 30 milligrams
- Oregon grape (berberine): 70 milligrams
- Blend of Coptis root and rhizome, Chinese skullcap root, Phellodendron bark, Ginger rhizome, Chinese licorice root, Chinese rhubarb root and rhizome: 300 milligrams

Tricycline, from Allergy Research Group
- berberine HCL: 400 milligrams
- artemisinin: 60 milligrams
- citrus seed extract: 400 milligrams
- black walnut: 100 milligrams (hulls)

Oregano capsules, from Designs for Health
- oil of oregano: 150 milligrams

Biocidin (liquid or capsules), from Bio-Botanical Research
- bilberry extract (25 percent anthocyanosides), noni, milk thistle, echinacea (purpurea and angustifolia), goldenseal, shiitake, white willow (bark), garlic, grapeseed extract (minimum 90 percent polyphenols), black walnut (hull and leaf), raspberry, fumitory, gentian, tea tree oil, galbanum oil, lavender oil (plant and flower), oregano oil (plant and flower)

Berberine

Used for more than three thousand years in both Ayurvedic (a system of healing that originated in ancient India), and Chinese medicine, berberine is a compound present in various plants, including *Hydrastis canadensis* (goldenseal), *Coptis chinensis* (Coptis, or goldenthread), *Berberis aquifolium* (Oregon grape), *Berberis vulgaris* (barberry), and an Indian species called *Berberis aristata* (tree turmeric). Berberine can now be manufactured in the lab, often as berberine chloride or berberine sulfate. It has been traditionally used to treat bacterial diarrhea in China and has excellent antimicrobial activity against bacteria, fungi, parasites, worms, and viruses. However, in the last decade, it has become clear that berberine can do so much more than this. There are reports that it lowers blood pressure and blood sugar, treats cardiac arrhythmias, protects against cancer and dementia, reduces inflammation and pain, improves mood, and is a potent antioxidant that can quench free radicals.[20] Studies have shown that berberine reduces serum levels of pro-inflammatory cytokines in people with type 2 diabetes and cardiovascular disease and has been shown to be an effective option for treating ulcerative colitis.[21] It certainly seems like there isn't anything it can't do!

Berberine is an herb that is usually included in all dysbiosis protocols because of its ability to inhibit gut bacteria without being absorbed into the body. Its antibacterial prowess includes good activity against the following microbes: *Staphylococcus* (berberine is now being studied for use against the disease methicillin-resistant *Staphylococcus aureus*, or MRSA), *Streptococcus, Salmonella, Klebsiella, Clostridium, Pseudomonas, Proteus, Shigella, Vibrio*, and *Cryptococcus*. It also had some effect against diarrhea from toxin-producing *Escherichia coli*. The herb is believed to work by blocking the attachment of the bad bacteria to the intestinal lining as well as inhibiting cell division.[22] Not only is it safe for your good flora, but also researchers at Shanghai Jiao Tong University School of Medicine, in China, found that berberine restored good levels of lactobacillus and bifidobacterium in mice with dysbiosis.[23]

Although berberine has an excellent safety profile, don't use it if you are pregnant, because it can stimulate the uterus. It addition, the herb can cross the placenta and possibly harm the fetus. It can also be transferred through breast milk. Apart from these issues, there are no toxicities that harm your cells or genes when used in doses similar to or less than those in clinical studies. In the human clinical trials there were no deaths and only a few minor gastrointestinal side effects. Berberine does interact with some medications, however, so don't take it with the immune suppressant medication cyclosporine-A; Parkinson's disease medications that include the ingredient levodopa, like Sinemet; the cancer medicine cisplatin (Platinol); the blood thinner warfarin (Coumadin); or thiopental (Pentothal), most commonly used for anesthesia before surgery.[24]

Preliminary evidence suggests that taking 300 milligrams of berberine three times a day for six weeks is more effective than taking 150 milligrams of the stomach acid reducer ranitidine (Zantac) twice daily to treat the bacterium *Helicobacter pylori*, a stomach infection that is the number one cause of ulcers. But it is less effective in promoting ulcer healing in patients with *H. pylori*–associated duodenal ulcers, which are ulcers in the uppermost section of the small bowel.[25] Other studies have used up to 500 milligrams of berberine three times a day with no adverse effects, and it has been used safely in doses up to 2 grams a day for eight weeks in adults. It is likely unsafe for children, however. Although berberine has been reported to cause nausea, vomiting, hyper- or hypotension, respiratory failure, and the feeling of pins and needles (paresthesias), it's hard to find clinical evidence of these adverse effects in the medical literature. Other unwanted effects, including headache, slow heart rate (bradycardia), nausea, and vomiting, have been reported in both animals and humans.[26]

Several other herbs are also commonly used to treat dysbiosis. Here I will review some of them and the research supporting the effectiveness of each as an antibacterial, antiyeast, or antiparasitic treatment option.

Grapefruit Seed Extract

Grapefruit seed extract, which contains flavonoids with known biological effects—such as resveratrol, naringenin (high amounts in grapefruit), and hesperidin (high amounts in peppermint, oranges, lemons, and limes—has been shown to have good microbe-killing activity against bacteria and fungi and is believed to be as effective or even better than some antibiotics. In addition to its antimicrobial properties, grapefruit seed extract lowers levels of the inflammatory and free radical compounds TNF-alpha and NFkB. Other citrus flavones from grapefruit seed extract have been found in blood and body tissues after ingestion, indicating that it has a systemwide effect as well as an impact on gut microbes. Lactobacillus and bifidobacteria in the gut seem to be barely affected by grapefruit seed extract, and no severe side effects have been observed, making it an excellent option for treating dysbiosis.[27] In fact, it was found that grapefruit seed extract had a strong antimicrobial effect against *Salmonella enteritidis*.[28] The naringenin and hesperidin in the extract seem to be the active components. In a study of fifteen patients with the skin condition atopic eczema, 150 milligrams of oral grapefruit seed extract three times daily for one month reduced intestinal *Candida* spp. and *Geotrichum* spp., and slightly inhibited *Staphylococcus aureus*. All patients noted improvement in constipation, flatulence, abdominal discomfort, and night rest after four weeks of treatment.[29]

Researchers at the University of Texas Medical Branch, in Galveston, examined GSE to see whether it could be used instead of antibiotics to treat burn wounds. Remember, herbs need to work their magic without being toxic to humans, so it is important to look at studies that tested them on people, or at least human cells. The initial data show GSE to have antimicrobial properties against a wide range of organisms, making it what is called broad spectrum. And GSE works very quickly. Within fifteen minutes, it disrupts the bacterial membrane and kills the bacteria. The study used an extract called Citricidal, which can be found as a supplement either on its own or as an ingredient in other products. They found that GSE was lethal to ten different microbes taken from a burn wound in the skin, including *Enterobacter cloacae*, *E. coli*, *Acinetobacter baumannii*, *Pseudomonas aeruginosa*, and *Morganella morganii*—bacteria that can sometimes contribute to dysbiosis in the gut. This was an in vitro study, conducted in the lab in culture dishes, so we can't equate the dosing to humans, but the good news is that it was very effective at low doses that were not toxic to human cells.[30] Common doses of GSE range from 150 to 200 milligrams by mouth two or three times daily. However, because grapefruit juice can interact with many drugs, check with your doctor to see if it is safe to use with any medications you are on. (Although grapefruit seed extract is not the same as grapefruit juice, there are no studies showing that it wouldn't have the same effect. Therefore, it is better to be safe and avoid it if you are on medication that your doctor feels could possibly interact in a negative way.)

Arctostaphylos uva-ursi (*Bearberry*)

The leaves of the bearberry herb have been used traditionally as a remedy for a mild bladder infection, also known as cystitis. It contains phenols, hydroquinones, and tannins (ingredients found to be active against many microbes), as well as flavonoids, and has been found effective at inhibiting the growth of bacterial cells.[31] It is generally well tolerated when taken for weeks to a few months in traditional doses, but information from human studies is limited. The standard dose for treating a bladder infection is 250 to 300 milligrams up to three times per day, but when used in combination with herbal blends for treating gut dysbiosis, the dose is usually in the much lower range of 50 to 100 milligrams two to three times per day.[32]

Black Walnut (*Juglans nigra*)

Black walnut is also commonly included in herbal antimicrobial formulas to treat dysbiosis. Taken orally, black walnut has been traditionally used for diphtheria, syphilis, and treating worms. One study found that black walnut was effective in treating an antibiotic-resistant bacterial infection with *Staphylococcus epidermidis* when added to antibiotics.[33] A study at the Polish Academy of Sciences, in Warsaw, found that black walnut was effective against *Listeria monocytogenes, Staphylococcus aureus, Escherichia coli* O157:H7, *Brochothrix thermosphacta, Pseudomonas fragi, Salmonella typhimurium,* and *Lactobacillus plantarum.*[34] Anecdotal evidence, which relies on personal testimonials and not on rigorous scientific study, so it is considered far less reliable, suggests that black walnut has been used to relieve constipation and diarrhea. It is also rich in plant tannins, which have astringent properties and therefore reduce secretions and may relieve irritation. While capsules and tablets containing powdered black walnut are available commercially—usually in strengths of 500 milligrams and 1,000 milligrams—I have never used this herb alone. Like many of the herbs I've mentioned, it is safest to use black walnut as part of a broad-spectrum mixed blend so that the dose is lower: in the range of 50 to 100 milligrams two to three times each day. This is okay, since the herbs have additive effects and help one another work. Black walnut is not considered safe at the high dose for long-term use, which I would define as more than six months in a row, or if you are allergic to walnuts.[35]

Wormwood (Artemisia Annua)

Parasites can also cause a leaky gut and, as a result, systemic inflammation. Many people have parasites and don't even realize it because they don't always have gut symptoms, and often parasites are the underlying reason behind symptoms of inflammatory bowel syndrome, such as diarrhea and constipation. Tests don't always detect them because many parasites can live close to the wall of your intestines and therefore aren't passed in a daily bowel movement.

Because a parasitic infection can be hard to diagnose, I always recommend treating dysbiosis with an herbal blend that includes the herb wormwood (*Artemisia annua*), which has potent antiparasitic activity. This annual plant grows wild in Asia and southern Europe, but is now cultivated on a mass scale in India, China, and Vietnam.

Wormwood's medicinal ability to treat malaria is well studied and an important part of the treatment arsenal in countries with a high risk of that disease. Researchers at Poznan University of Medical Sciences, in Poland, discovered that artemisia extracts inhibited the growth of and killed an intestinal parasite called *Acanthamoeba*, whether it was living in a cyst form (protected within a shell of its own making) or free swimming. This is important because many parasites can turn into these cysts, which help them evade the immune system and treatment.

Parasites are more common than you think. Amoebas, for example, are a parasite that can live in the soil, air, freshwater, and saltwater, as well as in air-conditioning systems, drinking water, and swimming pools. They've even been found in contact lens fluid and bottled water! Artemisinin, the active substance in the wormwood plant, is believed to create free radicals, which help the immune system fight parasites. Artemisinin also appears to work against cancer cells, viruses, bacteria, and other parasites like flatworms and the protozoa that causes malaria, *Plasmodium falciparum*.[36] A more in-depth look showed that artemisinin also inhibited the growth of both bacteria and fungi.[37]

Artemisinin is generally safe and well tolerated. Various formulations have been used to treat malaria without toxicity, although you should never take it if you are pregnant.[38] Based on dose recommendations for the prescription antimalarial drug artemether (brand name, Coartem), a person weighing 132 pounds could take 96 milligrams a day. When you read a label on this herb product, it should say, for example, "150 milligrams of artemisia, standardized to 10 percent artemisinin," meaning that the dose would give you 15 milligrams toward your total for the day. My blends usually contain about 300 milligrams of artemisia, to be taken twice a day, for a total of 60 milligrams of artemisinin for the day.

Oregano Oil

Candida albicans is an important fungal pathogen, responsible for the majority of yeast infections. If it overgrows, it can contribute to dysbiosis and leaky gut. Its growth is usually controlled by your immune system and good bacteria. A history of antibiotic use can cause you to produce too much yeast. This can make you crave sugar and cause all the symptoms of dysbiosis, such as nausea, gas and bloating, and constipation or diarrhea.

Oregano oil is the most widely studied of all the essential oils for its ability to treat yeast. Researchers at the University of Eastern Piedmont, in Alessandria, Italy, found that oregano oil inhibited yeast activity more efficiently than the prescription antifungal clotrimazole (Lotrisone). It appears to damage the cell wall of the yeast and has been found to have antiviral, antibacterial, and antioxidant activity. Both oregano and thyme have high concentrations of phenols known for their effective antifungal activity, with oregano especially good against all strains of *C. albicans*.[39] Using the essential oil of oregano is more potent than the fresh herb.

In my practice, I commonly use oregano oil to treat yeast, either by itself or as part of a treatment plan that includes the prescription medications nystatin or fluconazole, or if these prescriptions fail to control yeast overgrowth. Scientists from the University of Tehran, in Iran, found oregano oil to be very effective against yeast that was resistant to fluconazole.[40] In other studies, oregano oil proved effective against a different species, fluconazole-resistant *Candida glabrate*.[41] In one study, participants took 200 milligrams of oregano with meals three times a day for six weeks, with no adverse effects.[42]

HERBAL BLENDS AND PACKETS

Apex Energetics, GI Synergy Packets (three capsules of herbs per packet)
- contains wormwood, black walnut, undecylenic acid, caprylic acid, barberry, olive leaf, garlic, uva-ursi (bearberry), catclaw, Pau d'arco, goldenseal, oregano, Chinese goldthread, yerba mansa

BlumHealthMD, Gut Cleanse packets (six capsules per packet)
- two capsules herbal blend that contains berberine sulfate, barberry (berberine), uva-ursi (bearberry), tribulus extract, magnesium caprylate, black walnut, artemisinin
- two capsules oil of oregano
- one capsule glutamine
- one capsule plant digestive enzyme blend (amylase, protease, diastase, lactase, glucoamylase, alpha-galactosidase, beta-glucanase, acid protease, phytase, cellulase, hemicellulase, invertase, lipase)

Treating Leaky Gut

Glutamine

Treating dysbiosis is the number one strategy for healing the damaged intestinal lining of leaky gut. Using probiotics to restore the health of the gut bacteria is part of the treatment for both dysbiosis and leaky gut, but other nutrients and supplements are also important. Glutamine, presently the best-known compound for reducing intestinal permeability, is one of the twenty naturally occurring amino acids found in protein and is the most abundant amino acid in the body. It is very concentrated in your muscles and an important food for all rapidly dividing cells in your body, especially your intestinal epithelial cells.

Animal studies have shown that a nutritional deficiency of glutamine results in major abnormalities in intestinal permeability in rats. In the lab, glutamine has been shown to maintain good epithelial integrity and to reduce permeability in intestinal cell cultures. In addition, glutamine supplementation has been shown to increase the intestinal barrier function in malnourished children and even in critically ill patients, where it reduced the frequency of infections following abdominal surgery. In low-birth-weight children, allergies were improved by glutamine treatment during the first year of life.[43]

A group of researchers at the University of Rouen in France studied people with irritable bowel syndrome, which has recently been linked to increased intestinal permeability. The goal was to determine the effect of taking glutamine supplements on tight junctions. In this study, researchers found that glutamine increased an important protein that regulates and repairs the tight junctions.[44]

Researchers at Fudan University in Shanghai, China, who studied the effects of glutamine in rats, found that it protected and repaired the intestinal lining from damage that normally occurs after trauma or major surgery, reducing the permeability and restoring the structure of the damaged villi. It also lowered the levels of inflammatory cytokines NFkB and TNF-alpha, among others, in the rats that received glutamine.[45] In other animal experiments, giving glutamine to mice that had an inflamed and leaky gut helped reduce permeability and reverse the damage.[46] Glutamine might also help remedy impaired gut motility, which can increase the risk of constipation, SIBO, and dysbiosis. Helping the bowels move well is an important part of treating the gut. Research involving cancer patients found that taking glutamine supplements helped protect the nervous system in their intestines from damage.[47] In terms of dosage, studies have used 3 to 20 grams per day. These were tolerated without side effects. I usually start with 6 to 8 grams per day for three to six months and then drop to 3 to 4 grams per day for another six months or until the leaky gut seems to be resolved, which can take one to two years.[48]

Curcumin

Turmeric is the name of a plant also known as *Curcuma longa*. The most important chemical components of turmeric are a group of compounds called curcuminoids, which include curcumin, a well-known herb used widely as a spice in curry powders and mustard. In China and India, it is also used medicinally to treat conditions such as dysplasia (the presence of abnormal cells) and diseases such as cancer. Curcumin has natural and remarkable anti-inflammatory properties, and studies have found it helpful in preventing and treating colitis.[49] The herb is also a strong antioxidant and supports a healthy and balanced immune system.[50] While curcumin has become well known for these properties and its ability to treat inflammation, it hasn't been studied as much for its effect on the intestinal lining. Here are the few that I found.

Researchers at Cangzhou Central Hospital in Hebei, China, treated rats with curcumin before an intestinal injury and found that it protected them from developing increased intestinal permeability and damage.[51] According to a study from the University of Arizona Health Sciences center, in Tucson, dietary curcumin increased the amount of lactobacillus in the colons of mice compared with those not treated with curcumin. Indirectly, this would strengthen the intestinal barrier by improving the activity of the good flora.[52]

Curcumin has been an integral part of the gut healing program that I have used to treat thousands of people in my practice. I usually use it in protein powders, but also in capsules and food, especially for the first few months of treating gut dysbiosis, because it is very soothing and reduces intestinal inflammation. It is also great at reducing arthritis symptoms, and I'll show you how to use it this way in chapter 7, "Food and Fire."

Other Nutrients

Resveratrol and zinc are two other nutrients that seem to improve the health of the tight junctions. In animal studies, resveratrol strengthened tight junctions and reduced intestinal permeability.[53] The presence or absence of zinc has been shown to impact the barrier, due at least partially to changes in tight junctions. Zinc also appears to have a protective effect on the epithelial cells, and taking zinc supplements has been shown to improve and even reverse alcohol-induced damage to the intestinal lining.[54] Researchers at the Lankenau Institute for Medical Research, in Wynnewood, Pennsylvania, found that zinc, quercetin, butyrate, and berberine all strengthened the barrier, and each had a unique effect on the tight junctions, suggesting multiple pathways by which the barrier function can be enhanced.[55] These results also offer additional support for the use of berberine in all dysbiosis treatment protocols.

MY FAVORITE SUPPLEMENTS FOR LEAKY GUT

- L-glutamine powder or capsules, from Designs for Health, Xymogen, Thorne
- Strengthen L-glutamine powder, from BlumHealthMD
- Glutagenics powder (L-glutamine, aloe inner leaf, and deglycyrrhized licorice, or DGL), from Metagenics
- Heartburn Tx (zinc carnosine, L-glutamine, glycine, N-acetylglucosamine, deglycyrrhized licorice [DGL], aloe vera inner fillet extract—contains shellfish), from Vital Nutrients
- Curcumin capsules or powder, Meriva capsules, from Thorne; UltraInflamX 360 protein powder, from Metagenics; Inflammatone capsules, from Designs for Health; curcumin, from BlumHealthMD
- Butyrate: best to add ghee (clarified butter) to food
- Digestive enzymes: Ortho Digestzyme, from Ortho Molecular; Vitalzymes Complete, from Klaire Labs; Complete Digestion Support, from BlumHealthMD

Real Gut Treatment Programs for Real Patients

All of the herbs and supplements that I have mentioned are a foundation of the Arthritis Protocol. For the past fifteen years, I have been using probiotics and herbal protocols for treating dysbiosis and healing leaky gut. In this chapter, my goal was to first show you that this is a scientifically sound approach; next, provide details about how to choose different products; and finally, give you examples of specific treatment protocols I used with the patients whose stories you have come to know throughout this book. Sometimes treating the gut requires only a few months; other times it takes a few years. It depends on how severe both your arthritis and gut damage are when you get started. If you begin with severe disease, as in June's case, you should be encouraged that you *will* get there, and you can use June's treatment to guide your program. On the other hand, if you are newly diagnosed with inflammatory arthritis or have osteoarthritis, you can follow how I worked with Robert. And if you're somewhere in between, the program I used with Robin is a good option.

June's Gut Program

It took thirteen months for June's pain to go away (while falling off the wagon a few times), and more than two years to finally heal her gut, but she is now at a point where she feels great, extremely energetic, and happy. She has shown such steady, solid improvement and resiliency that she hasn't had a flare-up in eighteen months. June is still dairy free, 95 percent gluten free, and 95 percent nightshade free. Also, because of this resiliency, June can indulge in her favorite treat—brandy, which has a lot of sugar—a few nights each week. While I know that two years seems long, shifting the inner terrain of your gut takes time and patience. The goal is permanent change and real remission, and if you follow this program, you will get there. Remember, for some of you, it probably took more than two years to develop arthritis, so you should expect it will take time for your gut bacteria to really change.

For the entire program, she took the following:

- Ther-Biotic Complete: two at bedtime
- UltraInflamX Plus 360 protein shake: one shake daily for breakfast
- L-glutamine powder: one teaspoon twice per day for year one and one teaspoon daily for year two; stopped after twenty-one months

Here is what she took for her gut dysbiosis:

First Gut Treatment
- Oregano caps: two caps twice per day for one month
- Tricycline caps: two caps twice per day for one month

Second Gut Treatment (Four Months Later)
- CandiBactin-BR: two tablets twice per day for one month

Third Gut Treatment (Three Months Later)
- BlumHealthMD Gut Cleanse packets: one packet twice per day for one month

Fourth Gut Treatment (Six Months Later)
- Tricycline herbs: two per day for one month
- Digestive enzymes: one taken with each meal
- Ortho Digestzyme digestive enzymes: one taken with each meal

Fifth Gut Treatment (Eighteen Months Later)
- Ortho Digestzyme digestive enzymes: one taken with each meal
- GI Synergy Packets: one packet of pills twice per day for six weeks

Robert's Gut Dysbiosis Treatment Program for Undifferentiated Arthritis

Remember Robert, the sixty-year-old attorney whom I was treating for high cholesterol, when he walked into my office with new inflammatory arthritis? His stool test showed me he had both bacteria and the yeast *Candida* in his gut. His arthritis resolved quickly over a four-month period after only one month of herb treatment for the gut dysbiosis and one month of a prescription medication for the *Candida*. Here is what Robert took.

First Gut Treatment

- UltraFlora Spectrum Probiotic, from Metagenics: one daily
- GI Microb X: two capsules twice per day for one month
- UltraInflamX Plus 360 protein shake: one shake daily for breakfast

Second Gut Treatment

- Diflucan prescription for yeast: 100 milligrams daily for thirty days
- UltraFlora Spectrum Probiotic: one daily
- UltraInflamX Plus 360 protein shake: one shake daily for breakfast

Robin's Gut Dysbiosis Treatment Program

Robin, a fifty-six-year-old woman with psoriatic arthritis, came to see me because she was having lots of pain in her wrists, knees, elbows, neck, and back for fifteen years, and had a history of psoriasis as well. She did very well with the following treatment program, and her gut symptoms and joint pain disappeared after three months of treatment.

First Gut Treatment

- BlumHealthMD Gut Cleanse packets: one packet twice per day for two months
- UltraInflamX Plus 360 protein shake: one shake daily for breakfast
- Ther-Biotic Complete probiotic: two at bedtime

Second Gut Treatment

- Biocidin capsules: three times daily for one month
- Ortho Digestzyme digestive enzymes: one per meal
- UltraInflamX Plus 360 protein shake: one shake daily for breakfast
- Ther-Biotic Complete probiotic: two at bedtime

Sherry's Gut Dysbiosis Treatment Program

Sherry's treatment for rheumatoid arthritis took a very long, circuitous route. She followed step 1, the Leaky Gut Diet for Arthritis, down to the tiniest detail but rarely took the recommended supplements for the entire first year because she was extremely anxious that they would make her feel nauseated, which did happen often. The take-home lesson is that everyone has a different path, but eventually you can get there. It took about eighteen months for her joint pain to go away and for her rheumatoid factor to drop to normal levels; this finally happened after she was able to do a full two months of gut treatment at full doses of both herbs and prescription medication.

First Gut Treatment

- The antibiotic ciprofloxacin (Cipro) to treat *Yersinia*, a harmful bacterium that we found in her stool test
- L-glutamine powder: one teaspoon twice daily
- ProBioMax probiotic (Xymogen): once daily

Second Gut Treatment

- Oregano oil: two twice daily for one month
- L-glutamine powder: one teaspoon twice daily
- ProBioMax probiotic: once daily

Third Gut Treatment

- CandiBactin-BR: two twice daily for one month
- Ther-Biotic Complete probiotic: two daily
- L-glutamine powder: one teaspoon twice daily
- Ortho Digestzyme digestive enzymes: one per meal

Fourth Gut Treatment

- Nystatin prescription for *Candida*: 500,000 units four times daily for two months
- Rifaximin prescription for SIBO: 550 milligrams twice daily for one month
- L-glutamine powder: one teaspoon twice daily
- Ther-Biotic Complete probiotic: twice daily

This treatment resolved her arthritis!

Fifth Gut Treatment

Sherry's arthritis was gone, but a stool test still showed dysbiosis.

- Tricycline: two twice daily for three weeks
- Oregano oil: two twice daily for two months
- L-glutamine powder: one teaspoon twice daily
- Ther-Biotic Complete probiotic: twice daily

Stool test and symptoms resolved!

Sharon's Treatment Program

Sharon had a difficult course of treatment because for most of the time we were working on her gut, she had terrible tooth pain, and it turned out she had an abscess that had been brewing for months. This kind of infection in the mouth can trigger ongoing gut dysbiosis and systemic inflammation, and so I am not surprised that it was so hard to help her get on track. But once her tooth was pulled, we started making progress.

First Gut Treatment

- L-glutamine powder: one teaspoon twice daily
- Biocidin drops: five drops three times daily
- Diflucan 100 milligrams: once daily for one month
- Ortho Digestzyme digestive enzymes: one per meal
- Ther-Biotic Complete probiotic: two at bedtime

Second Gut Treatment

- L-glutamine powder: one teaspoon twice daily
- Biocidin drops: five drops three times daily
- Ortho Digestzyme digestive enzymes: one per meal
- Ther-Biotic Complete probiotic: two at bedtime

Third Gut Treatment

- Biocidin drops in the Waterpik water flosser to treat oral micro-biome: ten drops daily
- Probiotic 225 for one month and then back to Ther-Biotic Complete: twice daily
- UltraInflamX Plus 360 protein shake: one shake daily for breakfast
- L-glutamine powder: one teaspoon twice daily
- Ortho Digestzyme digestive enzymes: one per meal

Fourth Gut Treatment: Focus on Repair

- Ther-Biotic Factor 6 Veggie Caps: 100 billion CFU
- Ther-Biotic Factor 4 Veggie Caps: bifidus-only probiotic
- L-glutamine powder: one teaspoon twice daily
- UltraInflamX Plus 360 protein shake: one shake daily for breakfast
- Ortho Digestzyme digestive enzymes: one per meal

Tina's Gut Treatment Program

Tina has a mild case of ankylosing spondylitis, requiring only Mobic when she overdoes it, and because she's very athletic, this happens frequently. Over the months that we worked on her gut, she was able to take less and less while she did more and more.

First Gut Treatment

- Glutagenics powder: one teaspoon twice daily
- Gut Cleanse packets: one packet twice daily for one month
- Ther-Biotic Complete probiotic: two at bedtime
- OptiCleanse GHI protein shake: one shake daily for breakfast

Second Gut Treatment

- GI Microb X: twice daily for one month
- Biocidin: five drops three times daily
- Glutagenics powder: one teaspoon twice daily
- UltraInflamX Plus 360 protein shake: one shake daily for breakfast
- Ther-Biotic Complete probiotic: two at bedtime

Third Gut Treatment

A stool test indicated that Tina needed more treatment.

- GI synergy packets: one packet twice daily for six weeks
- Glutagenics powder: one teaspoon twice daily
- UltraInflamX Plus 360 protein shake: one shake daily for breakfast
- Ther-Biotic Complete probiotic: two at bedtime

PART 3

Treating Your Terrain

My husband loves wine and collects different bottles from all over the world. While I don't share his enthusiasm—mainly because it gives me a wicked hangover the next day, with brain fog, reflux, and fatigue—I've come to appreciate wine and understand that the health and flavor of the grapes depend on the soil, a wine-making term called "terroir," or terrain. I love this concept because I believe that the human body also has an inner "soil" that includes all the fluids that our cells are bathed in and that the health of this inner terrain determines how well our cells, organs, and bodies function. A terrain filled with inflammation will promote disease and vice versa. The two most important factors for creating a healthy (or unhealthy) inner terrain are the foods you eat and the balance (or imbalance) in your stress system over the long term, not just this week or this month. In part 3, "Treating Your Terrain," we will explore different diets and how they affect arthritis, as well as the role that stress and trauma might be having in your joint pain—and illustrate, with stories of real patients, what you can do about this.

CHAPTER 7

Food and Fire

I devoted a large part of my first book, *The Immune System Recovery Plan*, to nutrition and using food as medicine to treat autoimmune disease—information that holds true for every kind of arthritis, too. This nutritional approach means eating foods that lower inflammation and avoiding foods that trigger it. After many years of using food as medicine and answering questions from thousands of people, at both the Blum Center and our online community, who have been following the program outlined in the book, I realized that there is a lot of confusion about what to eat, thanks to many online articles and books on the subject. Some of these have been written by my esteemed friends and colleagues from the integrative and functional medicine worlds, and the confusion comes from conflicting ideas and recommendations for food plans ranging from paleo, to vegan, to gluten free. Then there are the internet sensations touting quick-fix diets that are extreme, restrictive, and may help only temporarily. If I weren't an expert in nutritional medicine, I'd be confused, too!

My goal in this chapter is to point out that many of these programs have certain things in common, such as eliminating processed foods and sugar. These commonalities are probably why many of them successfully help people lose weight and feel better. By showing you the simple guidelines that most of these programs follow, we can lay out a simple, scientifically proven approach that you can easily live with, not just now but also in the future.

As you now know, inflammation is the root of all chronic illness, including arthritis, and reducing inflammation is our number one goal for choosing a nutrition plan. Instead of taking medication to shut it off after it has already manifested and is running amok in your body, the goal is to find the causes of inflammation before it has even started, thus preventing it in the first place. This is why functional medicine and nutritional medicine are often referred to as "upstream medicine." Food has the power to trigger inflammation directly via nutrients such as sugar and animal fats, or from the lack of omega-3 fats and antioxidants. It also has an indirect ability to change inflammation in the body because it alters the gut flora.

My focus for your anti-inflammatory diet is on what you *should* eat: foods that directly lower inflammation and foods that support good gut health. My goal is to explain why you should eat these wonderful, nutrient-dense foods by sharing studies on arthritis and diet and the research on food and gut bacteria. We will also look at many different popular diets that you've heard of and may have even followed at one time or another. What the best of these diets have in common is a focus on eating a colorful rainbow of vegetables and fruit, legumes, whole grains, and healthy fats, and avoiding or limiting sugar, processed carbohydrates, red meat, and dairy. These are the basic nutritional principles for reducing inflammation and the long-term goal of eating for prevention and wellness.

However, there is more to the story when it comes to autoimmunity and arthritis, because you also have a leaky gut. This means that you probably have food sensitivities because undigested food has been "leaking" into your body through the intestinal lining and triggering an immune response, which then leads to inflammation. For example, a Mediterranean diet is a good basic food plan. But it might need to be personalized for *you* if, say, you find that tomatoes trigger more pain and swelling in your joints. This is why, at the beginning of a treatment program for any inflammatory condition, we always start with some kind of an elimination diet (also known as an oligoantigenic diet) to remove those foods that are the biggest culprits. I call this food plan the Leaky Gut Diet for Arthritis. This is not meant to be a permanent way to eat, but a temporary one, lasting from weeks to months until the leaky gut is repaired; then these foods can be eaten again in moderation. While my colleagues and I might have slightly different elimination diets, some more restrictive than others, the goal is always to *remove* foods that may be causing you symptoms and then *reintroduce* them after several weeks or months to identify any food reactions: not only joint pain and inflammation but also gas, bloating, headache, fatigue, brain fog, or just about any new or familiar symptom. This is how *you* will determine your own food sensitivities and create a personal list of what foods to avoid until your gut is healed. I will explain how to do this in chapter 10, "3-Step Arthritis Protocol and Guide." Using food that continues to reduce inflammation in your body is the foundation of the Healthy Eating Plan that you will begin after your step 2, Two-Month Intensive Gut Repair, when you move into the Finish-What-You-Started Six-Month Program of the Arthritis Protocol—and what I hope will be a permanent change in your daily food choices.

The History of Our Food Supply

Some people wonder why today more people are allergic or sensitive to foods than our parents or grandparents were. This is because our food has changed drastically since the 1950s, leading to a pattern of eating that is now called the standard American or Western diet—one that has been proven to negatively affect our health. It doesn't appear to be a coincidence that the current epidemics of obesity and chronic inflammatory diseases such as autoimmune disease and arthritis have coincided with changes in our food supply. This has prompted a lot of speculation and research into whether these changes are responsible for our society's worsening health. Each day, Americans eat less fiber and gobble down more processed food and sugar than they did before. These foods have increased the number of calories we consume. Couple this with our decreasing levels of physical activity and it's clear why the number of people who are overweight and obese keeps rising. But these changes have also influenced the gut bacteria and are clearly one of the reasons that we find ourselves with an upsurge in diseases associated with dysbiosis and a leaky gut.

What's changed? In the post–World War II years of the 1950s, we began refining grains, so that by 2005, 85 percent of cereals consumed in United States came from highly processed refined grains. We also developed technology to create processed sugar and high-fructose corn syrup, and our food became filled with these ingredients. In addition, we developed the technology to process vegetable and seed oils, including solvent extraction, mechanized expeller pressing, and something called hydrogenation, a chemical process that enhances the oil's shelf life. These are typically labeled "partially hydrogenated oils" and have proven to be especially bad for us, increasing our risk of cardiovascular disease. This has taken fats that would naturally be anti-inflammatory and stripped them of their antioxidants, so they may actually increase oxidative stress in the body.

The quality of our meat has changed, too. Before this postwar period, cows grazed and ate grass. But then they were moved to what are called feedlots and forcefully conditioned to eat corn, which isn't their natural diet. Their body fat increased, which is good for their owners, who want to bring them to market more quickly.[1] And at the same time, the dairy industry exploded as the cows became domesticated and used for this purpose on a mass-market scale.

Scientist Loren Cordain is often called the father of the paleo movement, a nutritional approach that advocates consuming only foods that our ancestors ate during the Paleolithic era, when humans were hunter-gatherers eating mostly animals and vegetables. A professor at Colorado State University, Cordain studied this diet very carefully and created a list of foods that have taken over our food supply since the 1950s, including dairy, cereal grains, refined sugar, refined vegetable oils, alcohol, added salt, and seeds and plants that have been genetically modified (GM) and hybridized (one species mated with another to create a genetically "new" offspring). He concluded that these "new foods" are the root cause of 50 percent to 65 percent of chronic diseases in American adults. In 2005, the items on his list, which doesn't contain any vegetables, fruit, nuts, seeds, or legumes, made up to 71 percent of all foods consumed in the United States. Cordain argues that the chronic disease epidemic is based on the disconnect between our genes and our new environment. In other words, our genes were perfectly suited to help us digest and metabolize the old foods, and until they adapt to these new foods—which takes thousands of years—we will have more disease and death and infertility. Our genes just haven't had enough time to catch up.[2]

There are many health implications of these new foods because they are different in glycemic load, fat content, macronutrient composition, micronutrient density, acid-base balance, sodium-potassium ratio, and fiber content.

Glycemic Load

This refers to the ability of foods to raise your blood sugar level. (You can look up the glycemic index of a food online. I like the calculator from the University of Sydney at www.glycemicindex.com/food Search.php.) Studies reveal that a diet with a high glycemic load can cause diabetes and prediabetes, in addition to diseases that have an inflammatory component such as metabolic syndrome, obesity, coronary heart disease, hypertension, and high cholesterol, all conditions associated with osteoarthritis. In 2005 an estimated 40 percent of the average American's calories came from high glycemic foods. These included refined grains and sugar products as well as less-obvious foods like dairy and fructose. While full-fat dairy is thought to have a low glycemic load (skim milk is high glycemic), it contains compounds that can send insulin soaring just like white bread and fructose can. Chronically high insulin levels are damaging to the body because an excess concentration of this hormone in your bloodstream increases body fat, especially a harmful kind around your belly that not only expands your waistline but also pumps out inflammatory compounds such as leptin, which is associated with OA.[3] (We discussed this in chapter 3, "Osteoarthritis.")

Dietary Fats

When it comes to dietary fats, some are beneficial and some are harmful. Good fat eases inflammation, while bad fat fans the flames. Health-promoting fats include monounsaturated fats (olive oil, for instance) and polyunsaturated fats such as omega-3 (fish and flax) and omega-6 (from nuts and seeds). There are also a few good plant-based saturated fats, including avocado and coconut oil fat. Most of our disease-causing fats come from saturated fats in meat, milk, and cheese, and also from man-made trans-fatty acids, also called hydrogenated fats, found commonly in cake and frosting mixes, baked goods, and margarine.

I'm not saying that you have to give up these foods 100 percent for the rest of your life, but I want you to think about the quality of these foods, which is what has changed. Consider the following: *you eat what your food ate.* So if the steak you're having for dinner came from a cow who ate corn instead of grass, that meat will be filled with unhealthy fat because grass provides healthy omega fats; corn doesn't. Likewise, if the cow was given lots of hormones and antibiotics, which is standard procedure in most US feedlots, your steak will also contain harmful levels of hormones, antibiotics, and pesticides too. This is especially the case with dairy products, because cows concentrate these chemicals in their milk.

While the Leaky Gut Diet for Arthritis does not allow beef or dairy other than clarified butter (also called ghee), the Healthy Eating Plan in step 3, the Finish-What-You-Started Six-Month Program, reintroduces these foods to determine whether you are sensitive to them. If you are not, you can happily include some grass-fed organic beef and dairy in your diet in moderation (about once a week), following my suggested shopping list beginning on page 236. Grass-fed means these cows graze on grass *all* the time and organic means these pastures are pesticide free and the cows haven't been given hormones or antibiotics. Interestingly, ghee from these cows contains butyrate, which is healing for the gut and immune system.

Vegetable Oils

The two most important healthy fats are omega-3 and omega-6. When it comes to omega-6, there are some good sources, such as borage and evening primrose oil, and some not so good, like arachidonic acid, which is found in animal products. Back in the time of the hunter-gatherers, our ancestors ate two times as much omega-6 as they did omega-3. Since twentieth-century technology has allowed us to commercially process nuts and seeds and make vegetable oils, the ratio of omega-6 to omega-3 has gone up to 10 to 1! The omega-3s have become tremendously diluted in our food supply. Also, meat used to give us extra omega-3s, but now it doesn't because of the corn-fed cattle. Given that omega-3 is the most powerful anti-inflammatory fat, this change has helped foster our modern-day epidemic of chronic illness. Many studies, including those with arthritis patients, have shown the powerful positive effects of adding omega-3 to your diet.[4]

Macronutrients

These are substances our body requires in large amounts (as opposed to micronutrients, which are required in only trace amounts) and include carbohydrates, proteins, and fats. These have also changed as our modern diet has shifted from nutrient-dense fruits and vegetables to one that focuses on calorie-dense cereal and carbohydrates found in processed grains and sugar. The refined sugars, carbs, and vegetable oils we eat so much of today are lacking in vitamins and minerals. The lowest nutrient density comes from processed cereal grain products, something that most Americans eat daily. Studies have shown that the micronutrient content of the Western diet has dropped, resulting in populationwide deficiencies of vitamins A, B_6, and folate, and the minerals magnesium, calcium, and zinc. These deficiencies, which I find every day in my patients, put you at risk for developing infections and chronic illnesses such as autoimmune disease.

Fiber

Our consumption of this nutrient has changed, too. Whole foods, such as fruit, vegetables, legumes, and whole grains, are very high in fiber, whereas processed foods have little to none. Our ancestors ate 70 to 150 grams of fiber per day compared with our measly 10 to 15 grams. Studies show a clear link between a low-fiber diet and an increased risk of colon cancer. On the other hand, a diet high in fiber can help lower cholesterol, improve digestive health and hormone balance, reduce constipation and colon cancer susceptibility, and help the body remove toxins through the GI tract. It also makes you feel full, so a fiber-rich diet can help control your appetite and reduce the glycemic load of food because it makes their simple sugars less available. Fiber is also excellent for your gut microbiome, which is important for preventing and healing arthritis.[5]

Micronutrients

Since the mid-twentieth century, our intake of potassium has declined 400 percent, while our salt intake has increased by the same amount. This reflects our shift from vegetables to processed food, because a lot of salt is added to manufactured food. The result is an increase in hypertension, stroke, kidney stones, osteoporosis, stomach cancer, and asthma. Our food is also contaminated by everything from new food additives used in processed foods to increase their shelf life, appearance, and taste, to an increase in residue from plastic containers and packaging. When you eliminate processed foods from your diet, you will be reducing these harmful chemicals too.

Acid-base Balance

The change in our food supply and food intake of the past sixty years has also shifted the acid-base balance of our diet toward being acidic, when for optimal wellness our bodies work better when we eat an alkaline diet. What does this mean? All the food you eat, when it's digested, releases either acid or bicarbonate into your circulation. According to the acid-alkaline theory, a diet high in meat, dairy, and processed grain is net acid producing, meaning that when you metabolize these foods, your body's biochemistry generates a lot of acid. The opposite happens when you eat vegetables, fruit, and nuts, as these foods create alkaline (base) compounds, with legumes being neutral. Before we started eating cereals and processed foods, our diet was net base producing; now it is considered high acid. The potential health effects of a high acid load include osteoporosis, sarcopenia (muscle wasting), calcium kidney stones, hypertension, exercise-induced asthma, chronic kidney insufficiency, metabolic syndrome, and osteoarthritis.

Gluten and Gliadin

Last but not least, our food supply has changed because of hybridization, which has increased the gluten and gliadin protein content in our wheat and introduced genetically modified foods into our diets without long-term studies on their health consequences. Our food supply has also become contaminated with pesticides and heavy metals, such as lead from soil and mercury from fish, and there is convincing evidence that these toxins are associated with autoimmune disease and other illnesses. (I will talk about managing this when we review the Leaky Gut Diet for Arthritis in step 1 of the Arthritis Protocol.)

Given all of these changes in the food supply and the Western diet that appear to promote inflammation and contribute to chronic disease, including arthritis and autoimmunity, there are basic goals that every nutritionist and health provider agrees on, no matter which "diet" he or she preaches. Based on this consensus, I have created these five guiding principles that should be lifelong changes in how you view and choose food:

1. Reduce refined sugar, high-fructose corn syrup, and refined grains.
2. Improve the quality of fat by removing refined oils and hydrogenated fats.
3. Improve the quality of the animal protein you eat by choosing organic, 100 percent grass-fed and finished beef (make sure they aren't "corn finished," meaning they are given corn to fatten them up before they are slaughtered), free-range chicken, and sustainably farmed, low-mercury fish.
4. Increase fiber, micronutrients, and phytonutrients (substances found in plants that benefit human health) by eating more vegetables and fruits, and choose organic when possible.
5. Limit salt, food dyes, and preservatives (which happens naturally when you limit processed foods).

Review of Popular Diets

Now that you know the principles of food quality that should guide all of your food choices, let's take a look at the different diets and what we know about their health benefits. Though they differ in their recommended amounts of fats, carbs, and protein—they all include some or all of my five principles. Therefore, what they have in common might be more important than what makes them different. This brief review focuses on the diets with the most scientific support regarding their health benefits and those that have something to teach you as a person with arthritis.

Mediterranean Diet

The Mediterranean diet (also called the Med diet) has the most research behind it as a beneficial, well-balanced approach to eating that lowers inflammation and reverses symptoms of chronic illness, including arthritis. (I will share some of these studies later.) This approach to staying well or reversing chronic disease emphasizes healthy fats such as olive oil, vegetables, fruits, nuts and seeds, beans and legumes, whole grains, and fish and other seafood, with small amounts of dairy and meat. It also includes moderate wine intake and is high in fiber, antioxidants, omega-3 and omega-6, and compounds called polyphenols, which are good for the gut bacteria according to several studies. In many regions around the world, the Med diet is their standard way of eating and is associated with longevity and vitality. It is relatively easy to follow because it is a diet of moderation and consists of foods that are very familiar to most people.

Extensive research has linked the Med diet to improved cognition, a lower cancer rate, cardiovascular benefits, and favorable effects on cholesterol, insulin and blood sugar levels, blood pressure, metabolic syndrome, and oxidative stress. It also reduces death from heart disease and the incidence of neurodegenerative diseases such as Alzheimer's and other dementias.

Low-Carb, Low-Glycemic, and Paleo Diets

The low-carb, low-glycemic, and paleo approaches limit carbohydrates to some degree and increase protein and fat. Carbs include vegetables, grains, fruit, and, to a lesser extent, beans and legumes. Studies show that restricting carbs is an effective weight loss strategy; however, there's not much evidence that eating this way results in positive health outcomes over your lifetime. Carb restriction is not a diet seen in many populations around the world, which always makes me wonder if it is the way humans are supposed to eat.[6] The low-glycemic option is better than low carb because it focuses on the *quality* of the carbs, which encourages you to make better choices instead of eliminating all foods in this category. Restricting foods with a high glycemic index and/or glycemic load means that your diet includes minimally processed, direct-from-nature foods instead of refined starch and added sugars. Extensive research on the positive health benefits of this sensible, balanced low-glycemic approach shows that it can also help with weight loss, but it is better than carb restriction in its ability to improve insulin metabolism, control diabetes, and reduce inflammation and blood pressure. These results were seen in both adults and children, and the cardiac benefits were greater than those from a high-protein paleo diet.

The most extreme low-carb diet is the paleo diet, which attempts to replicate the dietary pattern of our Stone Age ancestors. There are many different versions, but the basic principle is to avoid processed foods, dairy, and grains, and to eat vegetables, nuts, seeds, and meat instead. Some versions of the paleo diet allow legumes or fruit, while others don't. Solid studies have concluded that this type of diet is an effective way to lose weight.[7] However, I have a few concerns about the amount and quality of the protein. As we've discussed, meat today is different from the meat that our ancestors ate. If your source of animal protein is from what I call toxic cows, then this kind of diet can be very inflammatory. However, if your meat is from healthy cows, whose own bodies are not on fire with inflammatory fats and chemicals, or from wild game such as elk, bison, and buffalo—similar to the food our ancestors ate—it's a different story. Importantly, if all humans decided to eat paleo, we wouldn't be able to sustain this on a global scale because we can't raise enough cows to feed meat to seven billion people! The fact that it is not sustainable on a large scale makes me wonder if it is really good for us.

Low-Fat and Vegan Diets

Low-fat diets were a big fad in the 1980s, and I remember my excitement over the news that I could eat fat-free cookies and cakes and not gain weight. (Remember SnackWell's?) This is a great example of how, as a society, we conducted our own scientific experiments on ourselves without realizing it. By replacing fat with sugar and processed fat-free foods, America got . . . fat! Clearly this is not a healthy diet, but the question remains: Are there health benefits to following a low-fat vegetarian or vegan diet? "Low fat" is defined as a diet where 20 percent or less of the calories come from fat, compared with the usual recommendation of 25 percent to 30 percent. Most of the research has focused on low-fat diets and their positive effect on cholesterol and cardiovascular disease.

Low-fat diets are found in traditional Asian cultures, which focus on vegetables and vegetable protein instead of animal protein, and little processed food. Because large populations around the world eat this way, there is very extensive research on its health benefits, such as weight loss and reduced risks of cardiac disease and cancer. For people who have had a heart attack, its ability to reduce the chances of suffering another was equal to the Med diet (which is filled with lots of healthy fat). This suggests that the quality of fat is what matters and that avoiding all inflammatory fat derived from animals is probably what delivers the health benefits.

Vegan diets tend to be very low fat just for this reason: they don't include animal fats or proteins, and they emphasize eating plant protein like legumes, which are very low in fat. Also, vegans tend to be mindful eaters and live a healthy lifestyle in general, so they have less inflammation and body fat, lower blood sugar levels, and reduced risks of heart problems and cancer. That said, this dietary approach can be done well or poorly. I have seen many teens in my practice who became vegans and lived on pasta and junk food. Also, it isn't easy to get all your nutrients, especially protein, on a vegan diet. I know this from personal experience, because I followed this food plan for several years right before I was diagnosed with Hashimoto's thyroiditis in my late thirties. You need to be an "intentional vegan," focusing on vegetables and whole grains and making sure to find and eat legumes of all kinds every day to get enough protein. If you do, then this is a very sound way to eat and has clear health benefits. Still, you will need to get some select nutrients from supplements, such as vitamins D and B_{12}, and omega-3 fatty acids.

Alkaline Diet

An alkaline diet is very different from the modern Western diet, which is based on animal and cereal products, and generates excessive levels of acid in the body that is not balanced by fruits and vegetables. This is believed to cause a chronic, lifelong imbalance in the body called metabolic acidosis. When there is extra acid in the body, the kidneys must work overtime to help the body excrete it, which results in more acid in your urine, which increases your risk of kidney stones—especially uric acid stones. In addition, because the body also excretes more calcium and other base compounds to balance the acid, adherents of this diet see an increase in calcium stone formation, too. This calcium loss increases your risk of osteoporosis. Metabolic acidosis can cause insulin resistance and may increase your risk of diabetes, hypertension, and cardiovascular issues. This acidotic stress may play a role in the development of osteoarthritis, too.[8]

Metabolic acidosis also lowers the measure of acidity and alkalinity, or pH, of the tissues in your body, including your joints—a condition called tissue acidosis. All your tissues have acid-sensing ion channels (ASICs), which generate pain when they're triggered by an acid environment. Research has shown that the synovial fluid from the joints of rheumatoid arthritis sufferers has a lower pH (indicating more acidic) than that of people without RA, and the pain they feel is caused in part by ASIC receptors in the joints.[9] An alkaline diet can reverse metabolic acidosis, and it has consistently been shown to promote healthy bones, induce higher bone-building activity and bone mineralization, preserve muscle mass, and enhance toxin excretion. Also, in people who observe an alkaline diet, cancerous tumors tend to be less aggressive and less likely to spread to other parts of the body.[10]

When researchers at France's AgroParisTech university analyzed the protein and potassium contents of twenty different diets, they found that the ratio of protein to potassium determined the acid load from the diet. Foods with the highest acid loads were grains, meat, and dairy, and the lowest were fruits and vegetables.[11] To follow an alkaline diet, you simply need to observe the 70-to-30 rule: 30 percent of your diet comes from food that makes acid in the body after you metabolize it, such as meat, dairy, and grains, and 70 percent from alkaline sources such as vegetables and fruits. It's more about balance and less about restriction, so it can be a diet that you maintain long term. When you get started on the Arthritis Protocol, I will share some easy food lists.

Being aware of your diet's acid-alkaline balance seems sensible because it focuses on the functional aspect of the food you eat, not on calories. This is a reminder that all calories are not equal and that a piece of bacon will promote more acid and inflammation in the body than an avocado. Eating a more alkaline diet is a principle you can bring to any of the approaches I've discussed. For example, although the diets themselves don't instruct you to do this, you could emphasize eating alkaline and still follow a low-carb, low-glycemic, or low-fat diet. It would be harder to eat an alkaline paleo diet, but it *is* possible if you eat 70 percent vegetables and 30 percent protein. The Med diet is the only one that already provides a balanced alkaline plan, and maybe that's why it has repeatedly resulted in positive health outcomes for people who follow it.

In summary, can we say what popular diet is best for your health? I believe an alkaline, low-glycemic Med diet centered on eating healthy fats is the most sensible approach that you can maintain over a lifetime, while also following my five guiding principles for choosing food. This is the food plan in step 3, the Finish-What-You-Started Six-Month Program, and one that I hope will become your sensible home base.[12]

> Here are a few quotes from my favorite books from the author and activist Michael Pollan, such as *The Omnivore's Dilemma: A Natural History of Four Meals* and *In Defense of Food: An Eater's Manifesto*, both of which I recommend heartily!
>
> Eat food. Not too much. Mostly plants.
> Don't eat anything your great-grandmother wouldn't recognize as food.
> You are what you eat eats.
> Don't eat anything incapable of rotting.
> When chickens get to live like chickens, they'll taste like chickens, too.
> If it came from a plant, eat it; if it was made in a plant, don't.

Elimination Diet (Leaky Gut Diet)

Now that you know the basic principles of choosing healthy food from a more conventional perspective, we need to move into the world of functional nutrition, which looks at the direct connection between specific foods and how they can make your symptoms better or worse. What this means is that sometimes a specific food can cause an allergic reaction or a food-sensitivity reaction, usually because your body thinks this food is foreign and is launching an immune response against it. I have been talking about dysbiosis and leaky gut throughout this book, and it is widely understood that the worse your intestinal permeability, the more foods you will react to. These reactions can directly affect how you feel, so it is crucial to discover any foods that are doing this and drop them from your diet. Because the lab tests for food sensitivities are not really reliable, the best way to determine this is with an elimination diet, which I also call a leaky gut diet.

As a functional medicine specialist, I have been using leaky gut diets with my patients for more than fifteen years to uncover food sensitivities and remove these foods from their diets for several months while we work on gut repair. This is a great way to kick-start any functional medicine treatment program, and it is used regularly by me and my colleagues when we begin a new program with our patients. You will begin this in step 1, the Two-Week Jump-Start Leaky Gut Diet for Arthritis. Think of this as an experiment with two steps. First, you eliminate a list of foods. Then, after Step 2: Intensive Gut Repair (ten weeks from when you began), you reintroduce each food one at a time to see if you are sensitive to any of them. Bear in mind: this is not your permanent diet.

A leaky gut diet can target just one inflammatory food group—gluten, for instance—or it can include several common ones, such as gluten, dairy, soy, corn, eggs, and peanuts. It also banishes processed sugar, grains, and oils, which, as you have learned, is an underlying unifying principle for all successful food plans. Elimination diets have been well studied in children with attention deficit hyperactivity disorder, or ADHD, and I mention it here as an example of how they've been used with success to improve symptoms: in this case, focus and attention in youngsters.[13] A leaky gut diet is also the ideal way to develop your personalized nutrition plan, since you will discover which foods you need to avoid and which you don't.

Other diets are used in functional medicine for specific conditions. These include the specific carbohydrate diet for ulcerative colitis, the ketogenic diet for epilepsy and degenerative neurological disorders, and the FODMAP (an acronym for fermentable oligosaccharides, disaccharides, monosaccharides, and polyols) diet for small intestinal bacterial overgrowth (SIBO). They are very restrictive and, while appropriate for those with these conditions, are not meant to be adopted as a basic anti-inflammatory way of eating for general health and wellness. Because you have arthritis, and therefore might have an autoimmune condition, too, you will follow a very specific food plan for arthritis that also treats autoimmunity, supports the gut bacteria, and reduces oxidative stress and inflammation. This will be the focus of the rest of this chapter. After reviewing the research on the best foods for healthy gut bacteria and diets that have been shown to help improve arthritis symptoms, I will bring it all together so that you have a clear picture of how to use food as medicine to reduce your symptoms and reverse your arthritis.

Diet and Gut Health

When it comes to food and gut bacteria, the goals are to eat food that increases good bacteria and reduces the bad. Good bacteria make short-chain fatty acids and vitamins, don't make toxins, protect against pathogens, and help the immune system function properly. Harmful bacteria can make toxins, damage the gut, are associated with making cancer-causing compounds, and can metabolize environmental toxins into even worse chemicals.

As we review this information, there are a few guiding principles that I want you to keep in mind. The first is that the bacteria in your gut change with the food you eat because different bacteria are good at digesting different kinds of food. For example, *Bifidobacteria* are great at digesting fiber, and so when you eat fiber, they multiply and grow in number because they are *needed* for metabolizing the fiber you just ate. This is one reason why people who aren't used to eating vegetables can experience bloating and other digestive symptoms when they start eating these foods that are new to their gut bacteria, because it takes some time for them to grow the bacteria needed to help digest them.

Second, when looking at gut changes from the food you eat, probably even more important than the actual bacteria is the change in the compounds that are being produced by the bacteria. For example, the different kinds of short-chain fatty acids (we talked about butyrate, acetate, and propionate in chapter 5) and the total amount are important. Again, using fiber as an example, when you eat lots of fiber-laden foods, you make a lot of short-chain fatty acids. This lowers the pH in your colon, and the acid environment selectively kills bad bacteria while sparing the good. Accordingly, helping your gut flora turn out lots of these short-chain fatty acids is important for treating gut dysbiosis. On the flip side, when you eat a high-protein, low-carb (and low-fiber) diet, your bacteria ferment the protein instead of carbs and manufacture ammonia compounds that are harmful to your health. I will share those details in this section.

Finally, all of the studies that I reviewed make it very clear that diet can alter your gut bacteria and the compounds they make, but this change lasts only as long as the diet does. This means that in order to reap the long-term health benefits, you must commit to sticking to the eating plan for good, because otherwise your gut bacteria will just change again when you go back to your old eating habits. However, this does not mean that I recommend a strict way of eating for the rest of your life. To the contrary, the Healthy Eating Plan that I will show you as part of the Arthritis Protocol is a balanced Mediterranean diet with a few adjustments and something that you can follow easily.

Prebiotics: Fiber

A dietary prebiotic (not *probiotic*) is an ingredient that positively influences the composition and functioning of the gut microbiome, and these changes are beneficial for your health and well-being. Prebiotics are generally able to withstand digestion, and a large number of studies have shown that prebiotic food products, supplements, and ingredients bring about statistically significant changes in the gut flora. Some studies have also shown a reduction in bad bacteria such as *Salmonella* and *Clostridia*.

The vast majority of the bacteria in the colon are anaerobes and thus derive energy from fermentation of two main nutrients that escape digestion in the small intestine: nondigestible carbohydrates (fiber) and proteins. Nondigestible carbs include resistant starch, nonstarch polysaccharides (for example, pectins, arabinogalactans, gum arabic, guar gum, and hemicellulose), nondigestible oligosaccharides (raffinose, stachyose, galactans, and mannans), and undigested portions of disaccharides (lactose, for example) and sugar alcohols (lactitol, isomalt). The Western diet contains between 20 and 30 grams per day of nondigestible carbohydrates that are metabolized by gut bacteria species, including *Bacteroides, Bifidobacterium, Ruminococcus, Lactobacillus,* and *Clostridium.* These bacteria ferment the carbohydrates in the colon to short-chain fatty acids, which acidifies the colon and suppresses the growth of pathogens. They also improve intestinal motility, thus preventing constipation.

Inulin-type fructans are the most widely tested and studied prebiotics. They occur naturally in foods such as leeks, asparagus, chicory, artichokes, garlic, onions, wheat, bananas, oats, and soybeans, but only in trace amounts. As a result, it has become common practice to remove the active ingredient from these sources (especially chicory roots) and add them to more frequently consumed products, and you can now find inulin in cereals, baked goods, yogurts, sauces, drinks—even baby foods. Prebiotic supplements like inulin stimulate an increase in the good bacteria, especially those that make short-chain fatty acids. This lowers the pH in the colon, thereby inhibiting the growth of harmful bacteria.[14]

The role of nondigestible carbohydrates in the production of short-chain fatty acids is unquestionable. Based on its chemical and physical properties, dietary fiber can also be classified as soluble and insoluble. Pectin, oligosaccharides (including fructooligosaccharides and galactooligosaccharides), and inulin are soluble fiber. The fermentability of soluble fiber is high due to its capacity to dissolve in water, which allows for more effective digestion by microbial enzymes. Insoluble fiber includes compounds that make up the cell walls of plants and are harder to digest, including cellulose (the structural walls of all green plants), some hemicelluloses (bran, nuts, legumes, and whole grains), lignin (seeds, whole grains, bran, legumes, fruits, and vegetables), and arabinoxylans (cereal grains and grasses), which are also fermented but at a much lower rate than soluble fiber.[15]

Resistant starch, another valuable component of dietary fiber, is starch that escapes digestion in the small intestine and provides a source of fermentable food for colonic bacteria. It includes inaccessible starch granules locked inside whole grains and legumes, in addition to granular starch that is packed tightly, as in raw potato and other tubers, cereals, unripe bananas, and something called retrograded amylose, which is formed when a starch such as rice is cooked and cooled. It appears that resistant starch acts like a good prebiotic in the gut, too.[16]

Bacteria can also metabolize proteins, peptides, and amino acids from the diet, and it is estimated that approximately 25 grams of protein enter the colon of the average American adult each day. Unlike carbohydrate fermentation products, which are recognized as beneficial to health, it appears that some of the end products of amino acid metabolism are toxic and harmful, including ammonia, amines, and phenolic compounds. As a consequence, excessive fermentation of proteins—like what happens in a high-protein, low-carb diet—has been linked with colon cancer and inflammatory bowel disease. This is why it is better to shift the gut fermentation toward carbohydrates over the long term, because you will promote the formation of short-chain fatty acids, which have numerous benefits.[17]

Functional foods are those that are used because of their ability to affect some aspect of your health. Prebiotics are one example, as are natural functional foods such as apples, which have a dietary fiber called apple pectin. One study found that eating an apple a day increased several beneficial bacteria—among them *Bifidobacteria, Lactobacilli*, and *Streptococci*, with the biggest changes in the *Bifidobacteria*—and decreased potentially harmful bacteria such as *Pseudomonas, Clostridium perfringens* (associated with rheumatoid arthritis), and *Enterobacteriaceae*. Short-chain fatty acids increased, and fecal sulfide and ammonia decreased. This shows that the old saying "An apple a day keeps the doctor away" actually has a foundation in science! The effect is believed to come from the apple pectin, and other studies have shown that it has a superior effect on short-chain fatty acids than does oat fiber or corn bran.[18]

Prebiotics: Phytonutrients

Phytonutrients are the general name for healthy plant compounds. Within this are a group called polyphenols, which are believed to support gut health and are usually categorized into four classes: hydroxycinnamic acids, flavonoids, hydrolytic tannins, and oligomeric proanthocyanidins. Flavonoids, studied comprehensively for their role in preventing and treating diseases such as cancer and heart disease, are found in fruits, vegetables, grains, bark, roots, stems, flowers, tea, and wine, and have antioxidant, antiallergic, anticancer, anti-inflammatory, antimicrobial, and antidiarrheal functions. There are many kinds of flavonoids, many of which probably sound familiar, such as flavones, isoflavones, flavanones, catechins, and anthocyanins.

For example:

- Quercetin is commonly found in foods such as red wine, apples, onions, beer, spices, herbs, berries, and cocoa.
- Epigallocatechin is found in green tea.
- Hesperidin and naringenin are found in oranges.
- Apigenin and luteolin are found in beer, olive oil, aromatic herbs, and nuts.
- Genistein and daidzein, which are isoflavones, are found in soy products.
- Anthocyanins are found in red wine, grapes, berries, and pomegranates.

An estimated 90 percent to 95 percent of the total polyphenol intake can reach the colonic region without being absorbed. Researchers at Jinan University, in Guangzhou, China, found that both catechin and quercetin altered the composition of gut bacteria. Catechin suppressed Bacteroidetes, and both quercetin and catechin promoted *Bifidobacterium* spp.[19]

It appears that polyphenols and their metabolites can inhibit pathogens in the gut and stimulate beneficial bacteria, suggesting that they act as prebiotics. Therefore, the regular consumption of foods rich in phenolic compounds may beneficially balance the gut microbiota. It also appears that polyphenols are absorbed better when eaten with fat, but they may be blocked by protein and fiber and may not be well absorbed if you have altered gut flora. In one study, treating mice with antibiotics lowered the absorption of black currant anthocyanins. I find this fascinating, since my patients with dysbiosis often have high oxidative stress and low levels of antioxidants, even if they're eating a diet full of these foods. Healthy gut bacteria not only help absorption of these nutrients but also digest and change the nutrients into something called secondary metabolites. These might have even more powerful health benefits than the original compounds.[20]

Let's examine the effect of polyphenols on gut bacteria and health. Anthocyanins from cocoa and pomegranates stimulate the growth of *Lactobacillus* and *Bifidobacterium*. In rodents, pomegranate extract and apple juice were capable of increasing *Bifidobacterium* levels, while the *Lactobacillus* count increased after they consumed apple and red beet juice instead of water. Cocoa powder reduced the growth of Bacteroidetes, *Staphylococcus*, and *Clostridium*. In healthy adults, grapeseed extract rich in proanthocyanins, cocoa-isolated phenolic compounds, and isoflavone supplements were all able to increase *Bifidobacterium*, *Lactobacillus*, and butyrate-producing bacteria while inhibiting the growth of bacteria associated with gut dysbiosis in women. And there's good news for red wine lovers: studies showed that the moderate consumption of red wine by healthy volunteers over a period of twenty days increased the general phylum Firmicutes and Bacteroidetes and specifically *Bifidobacterium* and *Prevotella*. The *Bifidobacterium* population also increased after study participants drank a blueberry drink for six weeks.[21]

Specific Diets and Gut Health

It is no surprise, therefore, that fiber- and polyphenol-rich diets have a positive effect on gut health. This is supported by studies showing that a vegetarian diet is associated with increased short-chain fatty acids that can inhibit growth of less desirable bacteria such as *Enterobacteriaceae*.[22] In other studies, a Mediterranean diet clearly increases the levels of fecal short-chain fatty acids.[23]

Low-carb diets, on the other hand, exert a dramatic negative effect on gut bacteria. In one study, a high-protein, low-carb diet reduced the numbers of two bacteria that make beneficial short-chain fatty acids and increased the production of compounds thought to increase the risk of colon cancer. In another scientific investigation, there was a significant fall in *Bifidobacteria* numbers and short-chain fatty acids on the low-carb diet, but *Lactobacilli* numbers were unchanged. And according to yet another study, a reduction in dietary carbohydrates brought about a corresponding decrease in the abundance of *Roseburia* spp., *Eubacterium rectale*, and *Bifidobacterium* spp. Total short-chain fatty acids also fell in response to cutting down carbs. Finally, a low-carb, high-fat diet had a negative effect on the gut by reducing *Bifidobacterium* numbers, butyrate, total short-chain fatty acids, and frequency of bowel movements, as compared with the same number of calories consumed in a high-carb, high-fiber, low-fat diet.

Studies show consistently that low-carb diets do not support bacteria that make short-chain fatty acids, and this should be a warning to those following a paleo diet that overly restricts carbohydrates. While you might lose weight in the short run, this is not a good idea for the long term because of the negative effect on your gut health.

A diet high in monounsaturated fatty acids such as olive oil reduced total bacteria but didn't change the composition of the different species. Regularly consuming omega-3 fats from diet or supplements was associated with more *Lactobacillus* and improved epithelial integrity and barrier function, while consistently getting omega-6 fats by using processed vegetable oils was associated with lower amounts of *Bifidobacterium*. All of these studies highlight the role that food has for ensuring the health of your good gut bacteria. In the long term, eating gut-supportive foods is the optimal way to improve gut health—

better, in fact, than relying on probiotics. Yes, probiotics have a very positive effect while you take them, but they do not usually colonize the GI tract, so they need to be taken daily for benefits.[24]

Nonceliac Gluten Sensitivity (NCGS)

Before we move on to discussing specific diets and their effects on arthritis, one last word about elimination diets and gut health, with a specific mention about gluten. I wrote extensively about gluten and its role in triggering autoimmune disease in my first book, *The Immune System Recovery Plan*, so I won't cover it here in the same detail. Instead, I want to discuss briefly the recent new classification called nonceliac gluten sensitivity. We have seen an epidemic in gluten-related symptoms, including bloating, abdominal pain, diarrhea, fatigue, headache, anxiety, and cognitive issues. In the past, people with these symptoms have been met with disdain and disbelief by their gastroenterologists, who test them for celiac disease and then, because the results come back normal, insist they have no problem with gluten. Finally, this latest research provides ample proof that even in the absence of celiac disease, gluten can activate the immune response and also cause epithelial cell damage in the gut that goes undetected by the usual tests.

Previous studies have shown that people with NCGS had increased white blood cells in the gut lining, as well as elevated inflammatory and immune activity at the intestinal tight junctions and compromised intestinal epithelial integrity leading to a leaky gut. Although researchers from Columbia University Medical Center in New York found no immune response that was typical of celiac disease, people with nonceliac gluten sensitivity did exhibit an enhanced immune response to gliadin and bacterial cell wall components like serum lipopolysaccharide—the hallmarks of a leaky gut.[25] Because gluten appears to be so damaging to the gut, it needs to be eliminated as part of any gut repair program.

Diet and Rheumatoid Arthritis

An estimated 33 percent to 75 percent of RA patients believe that food plays an important role in the severity of their symptoms, and 20 percent to 50 percent have tried changing their diets to relieve their suffering. When people have many other health issues, such as diabetes and heart disease, it is common for their doctors to talk to them about the link between diet and these conditions. However, it's not at all common for medical professionals to have this discussion with arthritis patients. The goal here, therefore, is to provide the best advice on which diet is best for people experiencing autoimmune and inflammatory conditions, with pain as a central feature.[26]

As we discussed earlier, the Western diet is abundant in an omega-6 fat called linoleic acid, which is found in oils made from soybeans, safflowers, sunflowers, and corn oil. All four are commonly used in cooking and processed food. The body converts these fats into arachidonic acid, an inflammatory fat that is further metabolized into compounds called eicosanoids, many of which trigger the signs and symptoms of inflammatory joint disease: pain, redness, swelling, and loss of function. The omega-3 fat eicosapentaenoic acid (EPA) helps block some of these by inhibiting production of arachidonic acid and reducing inflammatory cytokines implicated in the tissue destruction of RA. Randomized controlled trials studying fish oil and rheumatoid arthritis have all shown improvement in pain when used in combination with medication. In these studies, there was a worsening of pain if the study participants stopped taking the fish oil.

Results of multiple studies showed that you need 2.7 to 4.0 grams of EPA plus the omega-3 fat docosahexaenoic acid (DHA) daily for at least twelve weeks to have a positive effect on symptoms. When taking fish oil was combined with a lactovegetarian diet (abstaining from meat products but not swearing off dairy), people's symptoms showed greater improvement than those who took fish oil or followed the vegetarian diet alone. This demonstrates that your diet is very important, and you can't just take fish oil supplements on top of an unhealthy Western diet and expect good results. Based on other studies, using fish oil this way can reduce the need for nonsteroidal anti-inflammatory drugs. I find these results very impressive because all of these clinical trials had recruited patients with long-standing RA. Omega-3 fats can also help prevent rheumatoid arthritis in people who eat fish for two or more meals per week compared with those who eat it less than once a week.

It is not surprising, then, that Mediterranean-type eating plans have shown improved symptoms because they are high in omega-3 fats from fish, nuts, and seeds, and also high in fruits, vegetables, legumes, olive oil, unsaturated fat, and antioxidants (providing lots of polyphenols), but low in red meat. According to a review of eight studies on dietary interventions, volunteers' pain scores improved on both lactovegetarian and Mediterranean diets.[27]

It is entirely possible that dietary changes might work by altering the gut bacteria. Researchers from Norway's Oslo University Hospital found that rheumatoid arthritis sufferers who had been on a vegetarian diet for a year had lower antibody titers to the bacterium *Proteus*, and this decrease was greater in those whose arthritis symptoms improved when they changed their diets. These benefits were also associated with changes in gut bacteria. Other studies have also shown a change in gut bacteria in those people whose symptoms improved when they went on a vegan diet.[28]

Researchers at the University of Glasgow, in Scotland, analyzed studies on the effect of diet in people with RA. Their findings: a vegan diet rich in legumes, fruits, and starches yielded decreased pain scores and joint stiffness after six months. Another study on the Mediterranean diet showed a reduction in CRP levels and DAS28, and an overall improvement in pain as well. Scientists also determined that these diets brought about the change in gut bacteria. They concluded that focusing on diet is a good way to treat dysbiosis and should be included as part of a treatment plan in addition to using probiotics and prebiotics in the forms of fiber supplementation and even considering the use of fecal microbial transplantation (FMT).[29]

Researchers at Ullevål University Hospital in Oslo, Norway, studied forty-three RA patients who were randomized into two groups. One group ate an uncooked vegan diet rich in *Lactobacilli*, while the other group continued their usual animal-based diet. Results revealed that the vegan diet changed the gut bacteria in RA patients and these changes were associated with an improvement in symptoms such as joint pain.[30]

Taken together, these findings suggest that dietary treatment deserves at least some of the credit for improving gut bacteria, and that Mediterranean, vegan, and vegetarian diets have all proved beneficial.[31] The Healthy Eating Plan, the long-term diet that I recommend in step 3, the Finish-What-You-Started Six-Month Program, is at its heart a Mediterranean diet with some added support for your gut bacteria, and it includes my five guidelines to choosing food.

One last word about elimination diets, since you will follow an elimination diet as part of step 1, the Two-Week Jump-Start Leaky Gut Diet for Arthritis: as someone with arthritis, you have to assume that you have dysbiosis and leaky gut. This is true no matter which type of arthritis you have, and this means that certain foods are triggering an immune reaction in your body—and maybe in your joints—because your leaky gut has been allowing many undigested food particles through the barrier of the intestinal lining. An elimination diet is a standard functional medicine approach to determine which foods are causing problems. Each person has a different pattern of food triggers, which is why an elimination diet is a key component of creating a personalized food plan.[32] Once you pinpoint your food triggers, these results will be integrated into your Healthy Eating Plan in step 3, and you will restrict those foods for six months.

Diet and Osteoarthritis

There is a strong connection between your diet and your pain level, which brings me back to my seventy-seven-year-old mother, Barbara, whose knee pain was at its peak after her walking tour of China. Within a few weeks of changing her diet and giving up alcohol, the pain had improved enough for her to take her dog on long walks, something she couldn't do before, and just a few weeks after that, she was pain free. Given the strong connection between obesity, excess body fat, and diabetes, and developing OA, it is clear that it is a metabolic disease, too, and not just structural. Therefore, to treat the foundational issue and to see true improvement, we must address the inflammation that is being triggered by your diet and perhaps by excess body fat and/or high blood sugar.

At Michigan State University in Grand Rapids, scientists studied whether a whole-foods, plant-based diet would improve pain and joint function in people with OA. For six weeks, one group ate its usual animal-foods-based diet, while a second group ate a whole-foods, plant-based-diet free of dairy, eggs, and animal foods. The second group's diet included unlimited amounts of vegetables, legumes, grains, and fruit, and small amounts of nuts and seeds. In the end, the plant-based diet group had significantly less pain than the group eating animal foods.[33] *The important takeaway is that you can improve your arthritis pain just by changing your diet!*

Other studies offer more evidence. Researchers at Australia's University of Sydney conducted an eighteen-month clinical trial of diet-induced weight loss in overweight and obese adults with knee pain. The participants, whose average age was 65.6, lost 10 percent of their body weight and saw a significant drop in knee pain, although there was no improvement seen on an MRI or X-ray.[34] While researchers were disappointed that the weight loss didn't improve the structure of the joint, this highlights the fact that body fat and weight can cause inflammation that contributes to your symptoms. That said, it also demonstrates that overweight men and women can help themselves feel better, function better, improve their quality of life, and reduce their medication by changing their diets and shedding some of that extra weight.

Summary

I hope that this chapter's review of changes in food during the past half century—along with the pros and cons of popular fad diets, explanations of how food and different dietary approaches affect the gut, and reviews of studies seeking to zero in on the best food plan for people with arthritis—has given you a deeper knowledge of nutrition in general and an understanding of the scientific foundation for the Healthy Eating Plan. The primary message is that an eating regimen that you can adopt long term should be a low-glycemic Mediterranean diet that is high in fiber, polyphenols, and healthy fats, and low in sugar, processed foods, dairy products, and red meat. It also includes fish and small amounts of lean meat. And even though both step 1, the Two-Week Jump-Start Leaky Gut Diet for Arthritis, and the Healthy Eating Plan in step 3, the Finish-What-You-Started Six-Month Program, are not intended to restrict calories, eating this way will help you lose excess weight and body fat (especially important if you have osteoarthritis), improve your gut bacteria, and reduce your arthritis symptoms.

CHAPTER 8

Traumatic Stress: Fueling the Flame

In the past decade, we have learned an enormous amount about the effects of childhood stress and trauma on illness later in life. The Adverse Childhood Experiences Study (ACE) is one of the largest investigations ever conducted to assess this connection. It is a collaboration between the CDC and Kaiser Permanente's Health Appraisal Clinic, in San Diego, that has followed seventeen thousand people since 1997. In 2009 this group published the first study suggesting a link between early childhood stressors and developing autoimmune disease decades later. The higher a study participant's ACE score, the more likely he or she was to develop an autoimmune disease. Rheumatoid arthritis was included in its findings.[1]

These results underscore the importance of looking at stress and past traumatic events in order to understand how they may influence your health now. In *The Immune System Recovery Plan*, I devoted an entire section to stress, outlining how it causes changes in the gut bacteria, intestinal lining, and gut-immune function. Over and over again, my patients and I connect stressful or traumatic events from the past or present to the reason they are having a flare-up or why they couldn't complete the program. The terrain of the body and particularly the gut are highly sensitive to the effects of stress hormones in early life and from current stressful events that cause them to be altered in a negative way. In order to really shift the body into a state of health—to create the conditions that allow the good bacteria and your immune system to thrive—it is critical to understand this and bring balance to your life with certain practices. All of your cells and every part of your being are affected by your emotions, hormones, and spiritual beliefs and practices.

Stress and Illness

Stress and Gut Dysbiosis

My Story: Triggered by Trauma

In *The Immune System Recovery Plan*, I shared the story of how I healed myself from Hashimoto's thyroiditis, an autoimmune condition of the thyroid, a large gland in the neck that produces hormones that regulate energy and metabolism. I had gone to my doctor for a checkup because my hands appeared sort of yellow (it turned out that my sluggish thyroid wasn't doing a good job of metabolizing the beta carotene from my diet), and blood tests showed the Hashimoto's. Briefly, this means that my immune system, which is normally the body's defense in the daily battle against infection and invaders, had turned on my thyroid, rendering it damaged and sluggish. I was surprised by this diagnosis because my only symptom was feeling a little tired, unlike the majority of my patients, who experience extreme fatigue, weight gain, feeling cold all the time, brain fog, hair loss, and difficulty sleeping. My doctor gave me a prescription to treat the symptoms (which I started), but I felt that popping a pill would merely mask my problem, not solve it. So, using a functional medicine approach, I also set out to determine the cause of my condition. I already knew that I had significant digestive issues because I had struggled with constipation and bloating since childhood and had terrible stomachaches and gastritis in medical school. One test revealed that I had a high blood level of mercury, and a stool test showed dysbiosis, which, as you now know, is an overgrowth of bad bacteria in the gut.

My treatment? An elimination diet, which meant avoiding dairy, gluten, corn, soy, eggs, sugar, red meat, and fish high in mercury, and eating an antioxidant-rich, vegetable-based, alkaline diet of colorful produce. In addition, I treated my high mercury levels with six months of supplements to support my liver, including protein shakes, antioxidants, and B vitamins, and I focused on treating my gut with three separate monthlong gut cleanses using similar herbal blends that I shared with you in the last chapter and glutamine powder for about two years. I also permanently changed my diet to focus on eating only whole foods and mostly plants.

Because functional medicine is a holistic approach looking at the whole person, including family, work, stress, and traumatic events, I knew that I needed to understand myself and how these things were influencing my health. I learned about the mind-body connection and acquired tools for relaxation, stress relief, and self-awareness. I began doing my detective work, gathering all the clues from my past and present, and realized that my stomach issues had started in childhood.

First, there was our family's diet of white bread, beef, fried food, and dairy—not at all unusual for the time. Second, there were the antibiotics I often took for chronic ear infections and tonsillitis. Despite their benefits, antibiotics can set you up for lifelong health issues by damaging the trillions of good bacteria that live in your gut. Taking probiotics can perhaps offer some protection against this imbalance, but in the 1960s, little was known about these "healthy" gut bacteria. Lastly, I realized that the dysfunction and fighting in my childhood home had filled me with anxiety. I vividly recall hiding fearfully under the dining room table while my father directed his explosive temper at one of my siblings. Thus, the mind-body skills I learned after my Hashimoto's diagnosis became a crucial part of my daily life and helped me to heal at the deepest level.

Within a year of beginning my self-prescribed functional medicine program, I was cured of Hashimoto's. This means that the overzealous antibodies that had been attacking my thyroid were gone, and my immune system was functioning properly. Within two years, all the mercury was out of my system, and my liver was well nourished and doing a great job of removing toxins from my body. My digestive issues were solved, and stool testing showed that my gut bacteria were repaired and in balance. I was sleeping well and practicing meditation, which kept my stress system in balance, and my thyroid was doing a good job of making its hormones, requiring only a tiny bit of prescription thyroid hormone replacement medication for support.

For five years, I maintained this strong state of health and kept these systems functioning well by exercising regularly, avoiding gluten and dairy (I had digestive symptoms and brain fog when I ate them), and taking a daily probiotic. Doing yoga, journaling, daily meditation, and taking long walks in nature without my phone helped me to manage the stress that comes with being a working, married mother of three children. With one son in middle school and two in high school, stress was par for the parenting course. Yes, there were several last-minute, late-night science projects, snowy car wrecks, emergency phone calls at one o'clock in the morning—a few from the local police station—and my children's stress from schoolwork and the college application process, but I handled it all pretty well.

For the first time, my life felt balanced. *I* felt balanced. (That therapeutic journey played a crucial role in creating the approach that I outlined in my first book, the bestselling *The Immune System Recovery Plan*.) But then, beginning in 2010, life intervened with not one but two major, devastating events.

First, there was my nineteen-year-old son's serious skateboarding accident that caused a terrible traumatic brain injury and the weeks, months, and years of angst as my son struggled to regain all of his functionality, which I described earlier in the book. But the trauma didn't stop there. Of course, this was hardest on him, but it also took an enormous toll on me and the rest of the family. Today he has recovered 100 percent, but it was a long road. Also, the same year as his accident, I was in the process of opening the Blum Center for Health and was setting out to write my first book. Therefore, the year following his accident, during the week, I worked full-time seeing patients and running the health center; on the weekends, I wrote;

and in between I fretted and tried to manage my son's recovery, even though he had gone back to school in Colorado. Writing the book, I was excited about the information that I wanted to share, so this was another form of good stress. I thrive on getting things done and felt very productive and happy. But I was *busy*. Because my schedule was jam-packed, and I was in a hurry to get to my desk in the mornings, I stopped meditating. For years, this mind-body technique was a way for me to relax both mentally and physically. It was the ideal antidote to stress because it helped balance all my hormones. It was also a way to sit quietly, check in with myself, and allow my true emotions to bubble up to the surface. This kind of awareness helps release strong emotional feelings so that they don't translate into internal stress that can adversely impact your terrain. It took me about six intense months to finish the book, and that meant six months where my soothing meditation practice fell by the wayside. And *that* meant that stress started to affect my digestion again. I also fell off the dietary wagon and began eating small amounts of dairy and gluten and drinking more alcohol and coffee, and my regimen of exercise, yoga, and long nature walks became less and less frequent.

Unfortunately, this wasn't the only trauma in my life. My seventy-seven-year-old father died suddenly of a massive stroke, a shocking experience for my entire family. His sudden death was traumatic enough but was only made worse by the subsequent conflict among my mother, three siblings, and me. And I wasn't the only one in my family suffering. Our youngest son had a particularly rough patch after his grandfather died (with whom he was very close) and really struggled when he went off to college six months later. He ended up coming home and needed a year off from school to gather himself, and needed me more than ever. I shifted my focus to my family, and we all got through it together. But in the meantime, I forgot to take care of myself.

It took a few years for the dust to really settle from my father's death and for life to get back on track with my family. Eventually my mother, siblings, and I were navigating the world without my father, and my three children and my husband were happy and productive. To say this was hard is an understatement, but we got there. Even though I have come to know that these moments when everyone is doing well can be fleeting, I was very grateful. In fact, we felt closer than ever thanks to the many things we had learned through experience and with the help of family therapy during my middle son's accident, my youngest needing to leave school, and my father's death. So, since finally everyone else in the family was okay . . . I fell apart and got sick.

This is another thing I see so often with patients: people hold it together very well during a crisis. They are competent and get things done. But once the acute drama passes, the after-effects of stress appear as symptoms revealing that the physical body has been shocked and changed by the experience. My digestive issues were back, I had pain in three of my fingers when I bent or pressed them, and I had one finger that would swell occasionally. Initially, I brushed this off as just part of getting older. That was until one morning when I woke up with eye pain that turned out to be episcleritis, an inflammation of the eye that is usually simple to treat with steroid eye drops and doesn't put your vision at risk. "You'll be fine in a few weeks," the ophthalmologist assured me. But when that time passed, and my eye was still inflamed despite three rounds of the drops, he suggested I see a rheumatologist. This is because episcleritis is associated with rheumatoid arthritis and other autoimmune diseases.

Then a lightbulb went off. I realized that the joint pain I'd ignored was a sign that there was inflammation in my body, and I feared that I could have RA. Besides my own history of Hashimoto's thyroiditis, I have a family history of autoimmune disease. Both my grandmother and my cousin had lupus, and my father had Hashimoto's, too. I also realized that while I wasn't paying attention, the trauma and stress had been slowly damaging my gut and immune system, leading to inflammation that I could now see and feel. It reminded me of the story of the shoemaker whose kids had no shoes: my specialty within functional medicine is rheumatology, but I hadn't realized that I had developed this problem!

What was happening to me was just like the iceberg that I told you about. Under the surface, there was a deep imbalance in my body that I couldn't see. Now it had grown to a size that finally made it visible above the surface as arthritis and eye inflammation. And what concerned me most was that I had no idea how bad it was or how worried I should be. Eventually I figured it out and cured myself, but before I share my test results and treatment program, let's talk about how stress and trauma can slowly change your body until you develop a symptom that you can see, such as arthritis.

What Is Traumatic Stress?

Trauma and stress are real triggers for inflammatory diseases. We live in a go-go-go world, one where we rush everywhere—even to yoga class, hurrying up to relax. Most of us are overconnected and perpetually "on," which activates our stress systems. Additionally, the epidemic of learning disabilities, ADHD, autism, and other childhood health issues that appear to be related to environmental toxins and food have many parents in a constant state of hypervigilance and fear. This is something I hear every day from my patients who are parents and grandparents struggling with these issues. On top of that, many adults, especially men and women in their forties and fifties, are caring for aging parents in a society that doesn't seem to support or value our older generation, and, well, you see where I am going. It is against this backdrop of ongoing stress that we experience additional traumatic events that, while somewhat expected in the course of life, still blindside us.

So what is traumatic stress and what is a traumatic event? Traumatic stress is an extreme version of the stress response that your body has following a traumatic event. Your body reacts to something sudden and terrible in two major ways. The first is a nervous system response. Your autonomic nervous system is considered the "automatic" part of your nervous system because it regulates your blood pressure and heart rate among other things, without you needing to think about it. The sympathetic nervous system is the "on" switch and the parasympathetic nervous system is the "off" switch, and these are supposed to balance each other. The sympathetic nervous system fires up when you are stressed, and this part of your stress response is often referred to as fight-or-flight. The parasympathetic nervous system functions as the brake, helping you to relax and turn off the stress response so that your body doesn't get stuck in the on position. This part of the stress response starts in your brain and travels down through your nerves, releasing chemicals called neurotransmitters that stimulate different organs in your body such as your stomach, heart, and lymphatic system organs, where your immune system cells are maturing and developing. A fired-up fight-or-flight nervous system response can manifest as heart palpitations, excessive sweating, difficulty sleeping, and intense feelings of anxiety.

The second way that your body reacts to a stressful situation or a traumatic event is by initiating a chain reaction in two areas of the brain, the hypothalamus and the pituitary, that control your hormones, cueing the adrenal gland atop each kidney to release the main stress hormone, cortisol. Like many things in life, this stress response isn't black and white. Not all stress is bad. Nature gave you a fight-or-flight response because the nervous system it activates and the hormones it releases can help you to run away from an attacker, or prepare you to give an important presentation, or get up the courage to ask for that raise at work, or ski down a black diamond run. These situations are all called stressors. Normally, when the stressor is over, your heart rate returns to normal, and your hormones come back into balance. At least that's what is *supposed* to happen.

When your stress system doesn't turn off, your body is bathed in hormones and neurotransmitters that can damage your gut bacteria and your intestinal lining, and also affect your mood, sleep, and energy.

Eventually this can lead to increased levels of inflammation, too. In the world of functional medicine, we have been talking about chronic stress and health for many years, and step 2 of *The Immune System Recovery Plan* focuses on balancing your stress hormones. For almost twenty years, as a faculty member of the Center for Mind-Body Medicine (CMBM), in Washington, DC, I have taught people mind-body tools for relaxation and balancing the stress system. I shared insights and many of those strategies in my last book. Since then, I have come face-to-face with trauma in my own life and realized that I need to expand the discussion to talk about trauma and the role it plays in all of our lives.

I have worked with many, many people who have suffered traumatic events, both in my medical practice and as part of a Center for Mind-Body Medicine team that went to Haiti several times after the catastrophic 2010 earthquake there. I have seen firsthand how traumatic events can set off a chain reaction that can ultimately lead to illness. A traumatic event is something that forces your body into a more intense stress response than the usual stress that you feel from, say, being late to work, taking care of an aging parent, or not sleeping enough. This extreme response can feel like an overload that is almost too much to handle. For most people, this is a state of high alert where you experience an increased heart rate, a clenched stomach, a racing mind. Often fear and anxiety take over, and you can become hypervigilant, meaning that your body is primed and ready to react to the slightest trigger. On the other hand, some people's traumatic stress response causes them to shut down, becoming numb to emotion, withdrawing, and feeling depressed. This is called the "freeze response."

If you could recover quickly and turn off the stress response after the trauma ended, it might not be as damaging. The problem? Most people go into either high alert or freeze up and stay there for a long time—often months to years. Often when people experience a trauma, even though they may seem to be getting over it, they can easily be triggered back into the acute stress state by memories, dreams, a new experience that feels similar to the initial one, or a comment from another person. This is called post-traumatic stress disorder (PTSD), which means that it's easy to trigger your mind and/or body to have the same reaction that you had when the traumatic event took place.[2] For many people, PTSD can interfere with their lives and damage their mental and physical health. As you can imagine, this is very hard on the body, as well as on the spirit and on the friends and family around you who want to connect and help you.

We are all familiar with PTSD in returning war veterans, but they're not the only ones who experience it. After Hurricane Katrina devastated New Orleans in 2005, I joined the Center for Mind-Body Medicine on five different missions over two years to work with people traumatized by the hurricane and its aftermath. CMBM is an incredible organization that helps to treat trauma and PTSD at home, working with the military and on Indian reservations, and globally, in places such as Haiti and war-torn Gaza and Israel. My role was to facilitate small groups of about ten people for a period of five days. I led and taught mind-body exercises to help them understand what had happened and to begin to bring their bodies back into balance, thus treating the PTSD with tools such as drawings, movement, meditation, and guided imagery.

I learned so much from all these hurricane survivors who shared their stories with me. One of the most profound lessons was that human beings have a natural inclination to compare their stories. Many trauma victims believe that their trauma isn't a big deal after they've heard stories that seem much worse. For example, in New Orleans a nurse told a story about being on the roof of the hospital with sick and dying ICU patients and having to be part of the team that decided who would live and who would be left behind. Another woman in our group felt embarrassed to share that she had been date-raped when she was younger and the huge impact it had on her throughout the rest of her life. She found it hard to share because she thought the nurse's trauma was much worse then hers. But the point is not to compare your trauma. Whatever *you* experienced is just as important, relevant, and meaningful to your emotional and physical wellness as anyone else's trauma is to him or to her.

After my son's skateboarding accident, every time I went into a hospital or thought about him attached to a respirator, my heart raced, my stomach tightened, and panic took hold of me. Because I watched my son struggle for a long time, I was still being triggered by reminders of what happened. This stress eventually caused a shift in the terrain of my gut, which was part of the cascade of events that triggered my arthritis. It was only after many months of mind-body practices, such as meditation, guided visualization, and, one of my favorites, shaking and dancing, that the fear began to move out of my body.

This brings me to lesson number one: trauma is held in the body in a different way than day-to-day stress. As a result, the mind-body techniques and strategies that you need to treat it are sometimes more focused on using movement than the usual stress management techniques are. Although I'm a trained facilitator in working with trauma, it took me awhile to realize that my son and I both needed to be treated for PTSD.

Experiencing traumatic events is just a part of life. We all lose parents and siblings, some lose children, many get divorced or get fired from their jobs. The list of potentially devastating or upsetting events goes on and on, but you get my point. Even if you are lucky enough to bypass any major trauma, we all have worries and anxiety. This can be just as hard on your body, because even when you merely *imagine* that something bad is happening, your body experiences it as if is *actually* taking place. Studies have shown that if your mind is stuck in a loop of anxiety, worry, and grief (sometimes without your realizing it, as in my case), it changes the terrain deep inside you to a place of dis-ease. To unravel this, your mind needs to let go of the fear, worries, and stress. The best way to achieve this is with a mind-body practice that makes you aware of what you are feeling each and every moment. When you use these practices, you can catch yourself when you are triggered into a stress response. After working so closely with so many people, I am certain that addressing these feelings, helping to stop the triggering, and moving trauma out of the body is the only path for deeper healing and a permanent shift in your state of health. Native American tradition says that we need to "be like the buffalo and go through the storm to get to the other side because we can't go around it." In other words, it's important to work *through* troubling emotions, not avoid them, so that these feelings are released and can no longer damage your physical being.

In my work over the years, I began to notice patterns in what was causing arthritis symptoms and the common struggles my patients were having in their quest to heal. A thread that runs through so many of these cases is how traumatic stress—past or present—is a trigger for arthritis. How does trauma cause illness? The current understanding is that PTSD may trigger inflammation through a process that starts like the stress response, with overactivation of the stress hormones and the sympathetic nervous system. But then, when the body tries to shut off this system it turns the cortisol so low that it increases inflammation and inflammatory-related diseases. In support of this hypothesis, researchers from the Geisinger Clinic in Danville, Pennsylvania, found that patients who suffered persistent PTSD symptoms were more likely to develop an inflammatory disease such as rheumatoid arthritis.[3]

Sometimes the trauma occurs in early life, but the damage shows up long after, persisting into adulthood. Evidence of this is the ACE study that I mentioned earlier, which tells us that alterations in the body that happen during times of persistent stress and in the aftermath of trauma can have a long-lasting, even permanent effect, which can trigger the development of disease many years later. This is why issues that you are holding on to must be uncovered, talked about, and addressed, so that you can reverse and heal your arthritis and inflammation, creating resiliency and shifting the body into a deeper and long-term place of positive health. Many times, arthritis comes on after a prolonged difficult stretch of time. Can you remember what was going on in your life in the year before your joint pain started? Or can you remember having been pummeled by a traumatic event, and your health somehow changed after that? Being aware and putting together the puzzle pieces are part of your personal arthritis story. This is a huge step on the path toward healing, because once you identify the possible reason(s) you became sick and/or keep having relapses, or why you might not be getting better, you can do something about it. To illustrate this point, I want to tell you about Jorge.

I met Jorge when he was nineteen and suffering terribly from juvenile rheumatoid arthritis (JRA). He grew up in Haiti and had terrible digestive issues and food intolerances as an infant and a toddler. He developed severe joint pain and was diagnosed with JRA at the age of five. Aspirin alone helped him stay pain free until he was thirteen years old, when he had a big flare-up, requiring the prescription steroid prednisone to bring him into remission. At this point, the arthritis was mostly in Jorge's knees.

When he was fifteen, the catastrophic 2010 earthquake in Haiti changed everything. He had been in his family home, which stayed intact, but his mother was trapped under rubble in another part of Port-au-Prince for eighteen hours and spent three weeks in the intensive care unit. She survived, but this triggered a major exacerbation of Jorge's symptoms that required even higher doses of prednisone (25 milligrams), which he was still taking in addition to the NSAID naproxen when he came to see me four years later.

He needed crutches because his knees were so painful and swollen that he couldn't put weight on them. We treated his gut multiple times and changed his diet and also talked about the traumatic stress he'd experienced and the role it might play in his ability to heal his JRA. While Jorge continued to improve every time we spoke over Skype, we were struggling to get him off the prednisone, managing to drop the dosage only 2 milligrams every three to four months.

And then something wonderful happened: we had a Skype call, and Jorge looked healthier than I had ever seen him. He excitedly told me that he had reduced his dose of prednisone 5 milligrams since our last call and was able to go up and down the stairs without crutches and pain. When I asked him what happened, he told me he had started meditating every day, adding that it was the *only* change he had made. And Jorge was just twenty at the time! The mind-body connection is very real and very strong.

Numerous studies have found that faith can also help change your health in a positive way. This is often attributed to the belief that you belong to something greater. Whatever the reason, the mind-body-spirit connection and awareness are important sources of nourishment that have positive effects on your internal environment. Awareness is the first step of the program, so I suggest that you take the ACE questionnaire (see sidebar on page 172) to better understand yourself, and to discover the factors that may have caused you to get sick in the first place. The questionnaire will show you what the experts define as traumatic events, and my hope is that this will convince you that traumatic events really do matter.

I also want to share an example of how this plays out in the lives of my patients. Brenda was thirty years old when we began working together. She had been suffering with joint pain since she was fifteen and was finally diagnosed with seronegative rheumatoid arthritis at twenty-nine. When we first met, she had terrible chronic pain and severe fatigue. Brenda had been on the prescription medications methotrexate and sulfasalazine but stopped them six months before we had our first consultation.

She told me that she had an extremely difficult childhood. She was fearful of her father, who was emotionally abusive to her, her younger brother, *and* her mom. Brenda had a good relationship with her long-term partner. They were hoping to get married and have children in the near future, but she wanted to get well first. She had a long history of digestive issues, with many years of international work and travel and recurrent parasites, so it took us almost two years to really get her gut in healthy shape with normal stool tests. Throughout that period, her energy improved steadily, as did her joint pain.

Brenda felt well enough to go back to graduate school, but every time she faced an important deadline, she would get very stressed, with an emotional response that she knew was more intense than it should be for something like a due date for a paper. She would also start putting herself down. The stress would cause her arthritis to get worse. Wondering if she was suffering from PTSD from her childhood and feeling well enough to dig into that part of her past, Brenda decided to begin seeing a therapist who specialized in adult children of abusive parents. She felt that dealing with her childhood abuse would be the final piece in establishing a link between her PTSD and her rheumatoid arthritis, and in agreement, I firmly supported this plan. Addressing this issue was especially crucial because she wanted to have this awareness not only for herself but also to enhance her relationship and for the children she hoped to have one day. When I scored her on the ACE questionnaire, she was a 3; a score of 2 or greater is associated with an increased risk of autoimmune disease. This supports the idea that Brenda's PTSD and other emotional issues likely exerted an influence on her physical health as an adult. She had already been meditating daily, and I encouraged her to continue this, while adding psychotherapy to her treatment program. It is never too late to deal with trauma from your past, and working to heal this deepest part of herself will help Brenda reduce her inflammation as well. Although she's just at the beginning of this journey, I recently spoke to Brenda, and she's already noticing a steady improvement in her joint pain and fatigue and is feeling better than ever before.

ADVERSE CHILDHOOD EXPERIENCES (ACES)

Directions: Answer each question with a yes or no, and give yourself 1 point for each yes.

Emotional Abuse

Did a parent or other adult in the household ...

1. Often or very often swear at you, insult you, or put you down?
2. Sometimes, often, or very often act in a way that made you think that you might be physically hurt?

Physical Abuse

Did a parent or other adult in the household ...

1. Often or very often push, grab, slap, or throw something at you?
2. Ever hit you so hard that you had marks or were injured?

Sexual Abuse

Did an adult or person at least five years older ever ...

1. Touch or fondle you in a sexual way?
2. Have you touch his or her body in a sexual way?
3. Attempt oral, anal, or vaginal intercourse with you?
4. Actually have oral, anal, or vaginal intercourse with you?

Substance Abuse in the Household

1. Did you live with anyone who was a problem drinker or alcoholic?
2. Did you live with anyone who used street drugs?

Mental Illness in the Household

1. Was a household member depressed or mentally ill?
2. Did a household member attempt suicide?

Mother Treated Violently

Was your mother or stepmother ...

1. Sometimes, often, or very often pushed, grabbed, slapped, or had something thrown at her?

2. Sometimes, often, or very often kicked, bitten, hit with a fist, or hit with something hard?
3. Were you ever hit repeatedly for at least a few minutes?
4. Ever threatened with or hurt by a knife or gun?

Incarcerated Household Member

1. Did a household member go to prison?

Parental Separation or Divorce

1. Were your parents ever separated or divorced?

Add up your score: a total of 2 or greater indicates that you have an increased risk of chronic illness, including autoimmune disease.

It isn't clear exactly why children who suffered trauma face such a high risk of inflammatory and chronic diseases later in life. One theory is that people with these experiences are more likely to engage in unhealthy behaviors such as smoking tobacco, poor dietary habits, and substance use, which are probably coping mechanisms. However, another reason could be that many of them have untreated post-traumatic stress disorder. Researchers from several institutions— the University of California, San Francisco; San Francisco Veteran's Affairs Medical Center and Northern California Institute for Research and Education; and Columbia University Medical Center— studied 735 military men and women with a current or past diagnosis of PTSD. The participants with current PTSD symptoms had significantly higher hsCRP (high-sensitivity C-reactive protein, a blood test that is considered a good marker for inflammation), and white blood cells (immune cells, a blood test that when high suggests an activated immune system), than did patients with no history of PTSD and those who had been treated for PTSD in the past and no longer had symptoms.[4] These results suggest that once the PTSD is treated, there should be less risk of disease in the body. This is good news!

From my clinical experience and understanding of the research, it's clear that traumatic events in the distant and recent past, as well as chronic or acute stress, can influence your current health and might be one of the root causes of the inflammation that is driving your arthritis or preventing you from full recovery. The first step is to become aware of this connection; the next is to do something about it. Fortunately, as was shown in the large clinical trial cited above, once the traumatic stress is treated, it will no longer have a harmful effect on your body. You don't have to let the past continue to define who you are and impair your health. With the right tools, you can change this pattern, and I will show you how in step 3, the Finish-What-You-Started Six-Month Program.

PART 4

The Blum Center 3-Step Arthritis Protocol

Now that you understand the roles that food, stress, trauma, and your gut health play in triggering arthritis and fueling the fire of pain and inflammation, it is time to put it all together into a treatment program that can reverse this whole process by helping you heal at the deepest places in your body. To do this, I share the exact program I used for myself, down to the smallest detail. It's just like the one I use with my patients.

However, as you may have noticed, all the programs follow the Arthritis Protocol but have slight variations. For instance, I treat dysbiosis with herbs, but which ones, and how often, and for how long can vary. Each patient's program is tailored to his or her circumstances. For example, some patients have no problem swallowing large pills, while others find this difficult. Or, although everyone is prescribed glutamine for leaky gut, some people prefer to take their supplements as powders that are easily mixed with water or put in a smoothie, while others opt for capsules. Allowing you to see these many options is why I've shared so many stories and detailed individual programs with you. My own story and my personal program will show how I implemented the Arthritis Protocol for myself. Hopefully, this will help you see that this is a very manageable program, and you can do it, too. I also hope that by illustrating the program with a real-life example, it will make it easier for you to follow.

CHAPTER 9

My Story: Putting It All Together

After ignoring my symptoms for a few months, I finally realized that I needed to fix my gut, address my stress, and work on my emotional well-being. The lightbulb went on when I realized that my eye inflammation wasn't just about my eye. (*Hello!*) There's a wise saying that a doctor shouldn't treat herself because there is a tendency to over-think symptoms and make impulsive decisions along the way. So even though I knew what to do, I turned to Elizabeth Greig, our nurse practitioner at the Blum Center for Health and a brilliant clinician who has worked with me since we opened. I wanted to have an unbiased expert weigh in on my personalized program. Elizabeth and I reviewed my symptoms, my story, and then all my test results, and formulated a treatment plan together.

Step 1: Two-Week Jump-Start Leaky Gut Diet for Arthritis, Supplements, and Testing

My first step (the equivalent of the initial consultation that I have with patients) was to run an array of tests to see if I had rheumatoid arthritis. As you know, arthritis can also be a symptom or complication of other autoimmune diseases and inflammatory conditions such as lupus, Sjögren's syndrome, scleroderma, dermatomyositis, psoriatic arthritis, and ankylosing spondylitis. You should ask your doctor to order these tests, too, which are easily done as part of a single panel during your blood draw and covered by insurance.

Happily, all of my blood tests were normal. However, I did find a mild-positive test result for something called a collagen complex antibody, which is not a disease marker itself but is believed to be associated with RA. This meant that I didn't have any of the inflammatory arthritis conditions that can be diagnosed with certainty. Instead, this left me with a diagnosis of undifferentiated arthritis, and a 30 percent chance of developing rheumatoid arthritis later on. So, while I was relieved that I didn't actually have RA, I was definitely afraid I was on my way to developing rheumatoid arthritis or something like it if I didn't act decisively. I also did a specialized stool analysis to look at my gut bacteria and a urine organic acids test, which can detect dysbiosis in the gut. These tests are available only from a functional medicine or integrative medicine practitioner and, while helpful, are not necessary to be able to follow this program. I share the information about these tests, and later on in my story I will also share the results, just to let you know how they can be used. Both of these tests take about four weeks to get results.

DR. BLUM'S PERSONAL WORKUP FOR ARTHRITIS

Tests to check for inflammatory arthritis, including RA:

My Blood Test Results That Were Normal
- rheumatoid factor
- ACPA (anti-citrullinated peptide antibody)
- ANA (anti-nuclear antibody)
- antibodies for Sjögren's syndrome, lupus, scleroderma, and dermato-myositis
- blood markers of inflammation: cardio C-reactive protein and erythrocyte sedimentation rate

- ANCA (anti-neutrophil cytoplasmic antibodies) panel, for diagnosing inflammation of the blood vessels, or vasculitis
- vitamin D
- celiac disease
- Lyme disease

My Blood Test Results That Were Abnormal

- intrinsic factor antibodies (autoimmune condition called pernicious anemia, which makes it hard to absorb vitamin B_{12})
- collagen complex antibodies; a possible early marker for RA but does not give a diagnosis. (Most routine labs don't perform this test. I did mine through Cyrex Laboratories, located in Phoenix: https://cyrex labs.com.)

While I was waiting for my test results, I immediately started the Leaky Gut Diet for Arthritis, a strict anti-inflammatory food plan and arthritis elimination diet. This meant no gluten, dairy, soy, corn, eggs, sugar, alcohol, coffee, food additives, preservatives, or dyes. It was clean, clean, clean. In addition, I ate organic as much as possible because pesticides can also damage the gut, and I avoided nightshade vegetables such as tomatoes, white potatoes, eggplant, and peppers. This food group is believed to aggravate arthritis symptoms.

When I say I was strict with the diet, I mean strict. Example? While visiting my in-laws in South Carolina, I diligently picked little pieces of red pepper out of my omelet, and on a summer trip to visit one of my sons in Colorado I stayed firm in my commitment to no alcohol—no easy task, given that a glass of wine would have been the perfect complement to watching the sun set over the mountains each night. My husband was very supportive along the way, but at one point he asked me when I'd be able to have a glass of wine with him. It was a good reminder that rigidly sticking to this plan has a trickle-down effect on those around you. This is why it's a good idea to discuss your program with friends and family *before* you start. Having a support system in place as you go through life is always important; during a health crisis, it's critical.

In the next chapter, "3-Step Arthritis Protocol and Guide," I will give you all the information and tools to follow the Leaky Gut Diet for Arthritis, but here I'll share a typical day of eating for me. Keep in mind that I have been eating a diet that is 95 percent free of gluten, dairy, soy, and corn for many years. By 95 percent, I mean that I eat this way at home, and, with a pantry and refrigerator filled with gluten-free, dairy-free, soy-free, and corn-free options, I never miss those foods. Then, when we go out to dinner, which is about once a week, I eat whatever I want. That said, around the time I developed arthritis, I had been traveling a lot for business and to visit family, so I had been cheating more than usual. Rebooting and cleaning up my diet, therefore, included being 100 percent "pure." I ditched chocolate and swore off almonds, which had caused stiffness in my fingers in the past. I even quit my morning espresso, an indulgence that I really didn't want to give up, but I did for two months.

For breakfast, I made a smoothie with my own Soothe protein powder blend, which contains curcumin, one of the most potent anti-inflammatory herbs. It has gut-healing properties and can reduce joint pain and swelling. The protein powder also contains glutamine and quercetin to heal my leaky gut, as well as omega-3 fats and ginger, which added to its anti-inflammatory potency. Each morning, I blenderized two scoops of Soothe with eight ounces of water and a cup of mixed frozen organic berries (blueberries, raspberries, blackberries). My goal was to make this as powerful in antioxidants and gut-supportive polyphenols as possible. Sometimes I added a handful of spinach or baby kale, too.

For lunch, my staple during the warm months of May through October was a large mixed organic green salad, including arugula, watercress, baby salad greens, and sometimes kale. I like to vary the greens to keep it interesting. Because I was avoiding nightshade vegetables, I needed to get a little more creative with my ingredients. I added radishes, celery, cucumber, jicama, olives, red onion, and scallions. For protein, I added beans. I usually make a big pot of beans every week, including adzuki, cannellini, and mung beans, and also chickpeas and lentils. Then I freeze half-cup single servings in the freezer so that I can just pull one out and add it to my salad before I leave for work. I also added some much-needed healthy fat by topping the salad with half an avocado, a tablespoon of pumpkin or sunflower seeds, and three to four tablespoons of salad dressing made with olive oil and lemon. I try to change up the vegetables, beans, and seeds every day to make my gut bacteria happy!

Because I have a late lunch in my schedule, I don't usually need an afternoon snack. But just in case, I always bring an apple with me to work. As for dinner, I eat home six nights a week and generally eat each of the following one night per week—chicken, fish, tofu, and eggs—and legumes the other two nights. Tofu night has been a staple in my house, and even my husband has gotten used to it. Actually, he will tell anyone who listens that he eats "like a rabbit" at home. But he does so proudly, especially because he is five foot ten, weighs 163, and has no health issues at fifty-six years old. He knows we are doing something right! He isn't a fan of beans or eggs for dinner, though, and on those nights, I usually make him chicken or grass-fed beef. When we go out to dinner, I eat fish. This has been my habit for a long time, and the only thing that changed while following the Leaky Gut Diet for Arthritis is that I had to give up the tofu and the eggs. Instead, I ate beans four nights per week instead of two.

The biggest adjustment was having to ban nightshade veggies from my stir-fry dishes. Instead of tomatoes, potatoes, eggplant, and peppers, I used different greens, such as spinach, all kinds of kale and chard, arugula, zucchini, broccoli, Brussels sprouts, asparagus, mushrooms, and every other organic vegetable that was not a nightshade. I also ate quinoa most nights, which made me happy, since I love it! For dessert, I had a handful of grapes or my favorite treat: a wild rice cake (or two) drizzled (or more like smothered) in olive oil.

It was easy to eat this way when I cooked at home, yet, as my patients usually tell me, it was challenging to eat out. Still, I found a way, because I needed to tend to my relationship with my husband, and for thirty years, we have gone out every Saturday night. I wanted to keep this tradition. Although it wasn't easy, I just passed on the glass of wine, stayed strict with no bread and dessert, picked the tomatoes out of the salad, and had a piece of grilled fish and veggies for my main course. The fear that I might develop rheumatoid arthritis kept me focused, and I stuck to the program.

I also added arthritis supplements. These included omega oils EPA, DHA, and GLA (gamma-linolenic acid, an anti-inflammatory omega-6 fatty acid) at high-enough doses to reduce inflammation (3 grams omega EPA/DHA and 500 milligrams GLA). I chose a liquid form that I added to my morning protein shake. I also took three additional supplements: vitamin D_3 (5,000 milligrams per day), anti-inflammatory capsules containing curcumin, and probiotics (multistrain, 25 billion CFU, or colony-forming units). For details, see the sidebar "Treatment Plan Started at First Visit" on page 183.

Tending to the Mind-Body Connection

For me, the mind-body component of the program had three parts: improve my sleep, start meditating again, and get support from others. As I began the Arthritis Protocol, I started making a plan for all these things. I knew it was best for me to get to bed at ten o'clock, but over the past several months, this had drifted to eleven. The body does important repair work between ten and eleven at night, and I've discovered over the years that the most optimal rest time for me is from ten at night to six in the morning. I have found this to be true for most of my patients as well.

Also, I returned to the relaxation practices that I had found so helpful in the past. Since my husband and I are empty nesters, I created a meditation space for myself in my son's old room, setting up an area in front of the window with my cushion and a tray on the floor to hold the spiritual objects that I have collected in my travels. This way, every morning I can just go into the room and meditate. I feel different just from entering this calming space that I created. If you don't have a cushion, you can use a favorite chair and make that your place to sit and breathe. (I will share resources for learning how to do this in chapter 10, "3-Step Arthritis Protocol and Guide.") I committed to a new routine: wake up, make green tea, and go sit for twenty minutes. I don't allow myself to check my phone or computer before meditation. My reward? The calm and mindfulness that I bring to the rest of my day. This helps me, but it also benefits my staff and patients. It's been a year now, and I am still doing this every day!

Finally, I sought out support from others. I found a therapist who could help me process and understand all the trauma, anxiety, and grief I'd experienced over the last few years and continue to enhance my relationships with my children and other family members. These are all the pieces that I put into place that I hoped would completely cure my joint pain and my eye inflammation.

TREATMENT PLAN STARTED AT FIRST VISIT

Supplements: Basic Arthritis Supplement Plan
- Soothe protein shake with antioxidants for gut integrity: two scoops of powder in one shake daily
- Probiotics: 25 billion once per day
- ProEFA omega liquid: one tablespoon in my shake
- Vitamin D$_3$: 5,000 milligrams per day
- Curcumin: 500 milligrams twice per day

Leaky Gut Diet for Arthritis
- No gluten, dairy, soy, corn, eggs, sugar, alcohol, and coffee.
- Avoid nightshade vegetables such as tomatoes, potatoes, eggplant, and peppers.
- Avoid food additives, preservatives, and dyes.

- Eat organic as close to 100 percent as possible.
- Focus on eating lots of greens and colorful vegetables.

Mind-Body
- Daily meditation practice
- Talk therapy sessions

Step 2: Two-Month Intensive Gut Repair

Two weeks into the program, I felt healthier than I had in a long time. The pain in my eye and my fingers had subsided, although not completely. My digestion and energy level, while not 100 percent, had improved. My sleep was much better, too, and I was beginning to feel well rested upon waking up in the morning.

I decided to start treating my gut with step 2, the Two-Month Intensive Gut Repair. A few weeks later, I got the results of my stool test and the urine organic acids test. As I'd suspected, they both confirmed that I had an overgrowth of bad bacteria in my gut, or dysbiosis. In other words, my gut was in bad shape. As a functional medicine expert who has studied and seen the connection between traumatic stress and dysbiosis, I wasn't surprised. But while I was busy taking care of others, I'd forgotten that this could happen to me! My gut bacteria—in fact, my life—needed to get back in balance. This sobering information motivated me to continue the two months of intensive gut treatment.

Twice a day for two months, I took an herbal combination of berberine, black walnut, artemisia, uva-ursi, and oregano oil. I call these herbs the "Gut Cleanse" because they clean out an overgrowth of harmful microbes. This is the most essential part of the Two-Month Intensive Gut Repair. Although some people have side effects from taking herbs, this is uncommon and didn't happen to me. In fact, most people feel better, with improvements in symptoms of gas, bloating, reflux, constipation, and diarrhea. Even though my stool test results revealed that my gut was a mess, I didn't have many symptoms to begin with. I see this in my patients, too, which is interesting because it means many of us are walking around with digestive systems that are out of balance, and we don't even know it! Also, as part of step 2, I added our Strengthen powder, containing L-glutamine, to my program to treat leaky gut and strengthen my intestinal lining.

By the time I finished the Two-Month Intensive Gut Repair, I had followed this program 100 percent for ten weeks. Thankfully, my joint pain was completely gone, and my eye inflammation and pain had also vanished, although my eye would redden easily if I felt stressed or didn't sleep enough. Now I could loosen up a bit and follow the program 95 percent of the time. This meant that I could have my espresso again and a glass of wine each week, which made me and my husband very happy!

MY STEP 2 TREATMENT PLAN

Supplements
- *Add* Gut Cleanse packets: one pill packet twice per day for thirty days. Includes herbs for gut cleanse, digestive enzymes, and glutamine.
- *Add* one teaspoon of L-glutamine powder to my daily shake.
- *Maintain* probiotics but take at bedtime while taking the Gut Cleanse packets.
- *Maintain* everything else from the Basic Arthritis Supplement Plan.

Diet
- *Maintain* the Arthritis Diet 100 percent.

Mind-Body
- *Maintain* daily meditation.
- *Maintain* talk therapy sessions.

Step 3: The Finish-What-You-Started Six-Month Program

It was September, and with the change of seasons, I felt I was transitioning too. The worst of my symptoms and the program intensity were behind me, and I felt hopeful because my physical symptoms were gone, except for my occasional eye redness. I decided to let go of any worry about my eye not being 100 percent and surrender to the belief that it would eventually get better if I followed the program. If not, the occasional redness in my eye might just be a permanent change in my body as a result of the inflammation that was there. Repeat stool testing showed improvement, so Elizabeth Greig and I decided that I didn't need any further gut cleansing. This confirmed the effectiveness of the Two-Month Intensive Gut Repair. It had removed the bad bacteria and started the healing process so that I could focus on improving my gut terrain in order to make permanent changes in my health.

The most important influences on your gut health are food and stress, which we've discussed throughout the book. Together, eating the right food, maintaining balance in your life and body, and having a healthy gut hold the key to creating deep and long-lasting resiliency and wellness. By following a lifestyle program that addresses these issues, you can shift your inner terrain—your inner soil—to one of sparkling, vibrant, good health that enables all your cells and tissues to do their best work.

Moving on to the Finish-What-You-Started Six-Month Program meant leaving the Leaky Gut Diet for Arthritis and returning back to the Healthy Eating Plan, which is the commonsense, balanced food plan that had been my home base since my Hashimoto's. However, I hadn't been following it very well when my arthritis started. I was able to add back eggs and coffee. Nightshade vegetables were still a problem, and almonds, too, so I kept them out of my diet. For my personal Healthy Eating Plan, I continued to forego gluten, dairy, soy, corn, sugar, almond, and nightshades. But instead of adhering to the plan 100 percent, this was now 95 percent of the time, which made it much easier to live with and not feel overly restricted and stressed.

That meant that I began to experiment with "cheating," which usually happened on Saturday nights when my husband and I went out to dinner. On one occasion, we went to an old favorite restaurant, where I had gluten, dairy, and alcohol all in the same meal. The next day, I felt pain in one of my fingers, and my eye was a little red and uncomfortable. But the symptoms were very mild compared with how severe they used to be, and after eating a clean diet again for a few days and getting a good night's sleep, they were gone. I was relieved that my symptoms resolved so quickly because this showed me that I was building resiliency. That said, I was still a little fearful and realized I had to be careful because I could slide right back to the beginning if I went completely off the program for too long. One day here and there every few weeks, my body could handle; but each time I had a reaction, it reminded me I wasn't quite resilient enough and needed to be vigilant.

I was making progress managing my stress as well. As part of my initial treatment plan, I set the wheels in motion to lighten my clinical practice, and my new schedule was starting to take effect. This created space for me to focus on my inner well-being. I was meditating almost every day but was having trouble quieting my mind and relaxing. I was practicing grief meditation and mantras to finally mourn the loss of my father and seeing progress in my relationships with my mother and siblings. But that wasn't enough. I was still tense, worried, and even a little anxious—an emotion that was not part of my nature or familiar to me. I also felt some stress stuck in my body, like a tightness lingering just beneath the surface.

I needed help moving that energy out and to fully address the effect of traumatic stress on my inner terrain at the cellular level. If I didn't do this, I was afraid that my gut, eye, and joint symptoms would return. I decided to try acupuncture, which is great at repairing and balancing all your organs, especially the adrenal glands, which are depleted by chronic stress. These eighty-minute weekly sessions worked wonders, allowing me to relax deeply and boost my healing. Because I was so worn out inside, it took about two months for my body to begin responding to the acupuncture treatments and two more months for me to feel the deeper stress and tension lifting and finally going away. At that point, my acupuncturist said that she could feel my body responding well to the treatment and getting better. I was excited and optimistic that my quest for health and resiliency was finally bearing fruit. But I was still only four months into step 3, the Finish-What-You-Started Six-Month Program, and, while I didn't feel daily inflammation in my body, my eye would still get red and feel irritated after I'd had any alcohol, reminding me that I wasn't quite finished with the program and hadn't yet reached 100 percent full recovery.

Another change I made was switching from seeing a family therapist, who had helped navigate the strained relationships after my father's death, to working with a therapist trained in somatic experience. This form of therapy aims to relieve symptoms of post-traumatic stress disorder and other trauma-related health problems by helping clients focus on the sensations they are experiencing in their body. ("Somatic" means "affecting the body.") With awareness, you can learn to use exercises such as breathing to alter your symptoms. I thought that this would help with the post-traumatic stress that I felt was still being held in my body from both my son's brain injury and my father's sudden death. I found a wonderful therapist for this, and after working together a few months, I had tools that I could use on my own to manage any anxiety from the old trauma, which happened less and less frequently. This last piece of my puzzle really helped me get through and over the traumatic stress. Finally, I felt that it wasn't in my body anymore. I did this and acupuncture at the same time, and together they helped me feel recovered. This was about six months into the Arthritis Protocol. After that, I stopped therapy but continued with acupuncture one to two times per month because it helps sustain me and keep me resilient while being an active, busy person who always seems to be doing too many things at the same time!

STEP 3: THE FINISH-WHAT-YOU-STARTED SIX-MONTH PROGRAM

Supplements

- *Discontinue* taking curcumin as a daily supplement; use as needed— for example, if my eye or joints felt irritated, which happened only when I ate a trigger food or drank alcohol.
- *Decrease* the dose of the EPA/DHA fish oil and the GLA omega-6 oil by half.
- *Maintain* vitamin D_3.
- *Maintain* one teaspoon of Strengthen L-glutamine powder in my daily Soothe protein shake.
- *Add* a daily multivitamin to my program.
- *Maintain* probiotics, to be taken with any meal.

Diet

- *Change* my diet to the Healthy Eating Plan, which is a *personalized* eating plan and followed 95 percent of the time. I reintroduced all the restricted foods from the Arthritis Diet one at a time to identify problem foods and then removed the food again if it triggered symptoms. I was able to tolerate eggs, coffee, and occasionally goat cheese.
- *Allow* occasional alcohol; about one drink per week.

Mind-Body

- *Add* weekly eighty-minute acupuncture sessions.
- *Maintain* daily meditation.
- *Change* therapy to the somatic experience approach.

I felt cautiously optimistic. My body had responded really well to the jump-start and intensive phases of the program and then to four months of deeper healing. While I was eager to be finished, I knew that unless I continued to focus on this and make some permanent lifestyle changes, the positive results would be temporary. This was a challenge because we were entering the Thanksgiving-Christmas holiday season, which is always hard to navigate when it comes to eating healthy and avoiding alcohol. Also, my family was going on a weeklong vacation to Mexico. I was concerned that I wouldn't be able to follow my program very well. And I was right. I went off the wagon with gusto. With holiday parties and other festivities, I had loosened up my restricted diet even before we got to Mexico and was eating trigger foods and drinking more than once a week. Then, on vacation, I enjoyed daily tequila (hey, it's Mexico) and splurged on foods that I don't normally eat, such as dairy (yogurt and cheese), salsa (which contains the nightshade veggie tomatoes), and tortillas (which contain corn). On top of the food and alcohol, on the last day of our vacation, we all had some unpleasant digestive symptoms, which turned out to be a traveler's stomach bug. I was worried that this would cause my symptoms to flare up, and, as I predicted, shortly after we returned home, I again experienced some redness in the white part of my eye and pain in one of my fingers. While I shouldn't have been surprised, I was certainly disappointed. I was afraid that the arthritis was back.

I believe that I initially got sick because emotional trauma and stress damaged my gut bacteria and caused leaky gut. After the Mexico trip, however, I think my gut was damaged from the stomach bug and all the alcohol. I decided to circle back and do another round of the Intensive Gut Repair, but for one month instead of two. This meant going back on the original strict, anti-inflammatory Arthritis Diet 100 percent and treating my gut with a unique herbal blend called Biocidin. After two weeks, my symptoms were gone, and after another two weeks, I returned to step 3, the Finish-What-You-Started Six-Month Program.

I learned an important lesson: that creating resiliency takes time, and it was much too soon for me to let myself go like I had in Mexico. Fortunately, it took me only two weeks to bounce back. But this is why I recommend the Finish-What-You-Started Six-Month Program for a minimum of six months, although some of you might do it longer.

I went back to following the Healthy Eating Plan 95 percent of the time. I feel great and symptom free on this easy-to-follow program. When I travel, my 95 percent drops to 80 percent, and as long as I go right back to the 95 percent when I get home, any symptoms are very mild and go away the next day.

TAKE-HOME POINTS

- Traumatic stress affects all of us and can damage gut function.
- Intense periods of unrelenting stress can eventually lead to inflammation and arthritis.
- After the initial period of intensive treatment brings improvement quickly, achieving resiliency and a permanent cure take time and a long-term commitment to the program.

CHAPTER 10

3-Step Arthritis Protocol and Guide

Step 1: Two-Week Jump-Start Leaky Gut Diet for Arthritis
Step 2: Two-Month Intensive Gut Repair
Step 3: Finish-What-You-Started Six-Month Program

Step 1: Two-Week Jump-Start Leaky Gut Diet for Arthritis

The first step to healing arthritis begins with repairing your gut, and this starts with your diet. Using food as medicine is a core part of our approach to treating arthritis and all inflammatory conditions. In step 1, you will remove foods from your diet that can trigger inflammation and learn which foods are healing, reduce inflammation, and support the growth of healthy gut flora. After changing your diet, you may see that some of your symptoms are caused or exacerbated by foods you eat routinely, and changing this will change how you feel. This is the exact program that I followed, and I know that you can do it too.

If you already follow a relaxation or mind-body practice, you should absolutely continue. I have chosen to introduce the mind-body program in step 3 so that you aren't overwhelmed by trying to do too much at once, because you need to focus on it with all your attention. However, you are certainly welcome to start it at any time!

TWO-WEEK JUMP-START LEAKY GUT DIET FOR ARTHRITIS AT-A-GLANCE SUMMARY

BEGIN: Leaky Gut Diet for Arthritis

- Elimination diet: remove gluten, dairy, soy, corn, eggs, peanuts, sugar, processed flour products, alcohol, tomatoes, potatoes, eggplant, and peppers.

BEGIN: Arthritis Supplements

- Omega-3 fish oil: 3 grams of EPA and DHA daily
- Omega-6: 500 milligrams of GLA from evening primrose or borage oil daily
- Soothe protein powder with antioxidants: one or two scoops in your daily morning shake
- Vitamin D_3: 2,000 IU (international units) daily
- Curcumin: 1,000 milligrams daily
- Probiotics: 25 billion CFU daily
- Multivitamin with antioxidants: two capsules daily
- Vitamin C: 1,000 milligrams daily

Suggested Schedule

Supplement	With Breakfast	With Lunch or Dinner
fish oil capsules	2	2
GLA capsules	1	1
omega liquid (an alternative to fish oil and GLA capsules)	1 tablespoon daily	
multivitamin with antioxidants	2	
vitamin D_3		1
curcumin	1	1
vitamin C	1	

(continued on next page)

Supplement	With Breakfast	With Lunch or Dinner
Soothe protein powder	1–2 scoops	
Probiotics	1	

The Leaky Gut Diet for Arthritis begins with an elimination diet, which means that you will cut out some inflammatory foods, including these common culprits: gluten, dairy, soy, corn, eggs, peanuts, alcohol, coffee, and sugar. Additionally, you will eliminate nightshade vegetables, which are known to trigger arthritis. Your comprehensive food plan is summarized in the table on page 202, and I have included shopping lists and recipes in chapter 11 to make this easy to follow. Yes, sticking with an elimination diet and changing what you eat is an adjustment. But in the Finish-What-You-Started Six-Month Program, you will reintroduce many of these foods, so this is more of a temporary experiment. Instead of focusing on what you *can't* eat, focus on the foods you *should* eat, because these will be part of the lifelong recommendations that I make in the Finish-What-You-Started Program. An improvement in your symptoms will make this all worthwhile, so get excited!

Five Guiding Principles for Choosing Food

First, I want to remind you about the five guiding principles for choosing food from chapter 7, "Food and Fire." You will see that my recommendations and food lists follow these principles, which are focused on the quality of your choices:

1. Reduce refined sugar, high-fructose corn syrup, and refined grains.
2. Improve the quality of fat by removing refined oils and hydrogenated fat.

3. Improve the quality of animal protein by choosing organic animals that are grass fed and finished beef, free-range chicken, and sustainably farmed, low-mercury fish.
4. Increase fiber, micronutrients, and phytonutrients by eating vegetables and fruits, choosing organic when possible.
5. Limit salt, food dyes, and preservatives (which happens naturally with limiting processed foods).

Food Focus

These are lifelong recommendations that you should begin now:

- Eat a rainbow of colorful vegetables and fruit every day. These are filled with antioxidants that support your immune system, as well as polyphenols and fiber, both of which feed your healthy flora.
- Include coconut products such as coconut oil, milk, yogurt, and kefir (a drink made with dairy or nondairy milk and cultured with bacteria). Coconut is filled with lauric acid and capric acid, two fats also called medium-chain triglycerides, which have bacteria-, yeast-, and virus-killing properties. It is also an easy-to-burn source of fuel that nourishes your brain and muscles.
- Include ghee, which is clarified butter. People with dairy sensitivities can usually eat ghee because all the milk proteins are removed, and it is pure fat. Ghee is filled with butyrate, a fatty acid that is critically important for the care and feeding of cells in your colon. Caveat: if you have a true dairy allergy diagnosed by your doctor, you should not eat ghee.
- Choose organic, non-GMO foods. Remember, everything you eat is the sum total of what the plants and animals were fed. Like foods containing pesticides and antibiotics, GMO foods can damage the gut lining, too, and eating them will work against the repair work we are doing to treat your arthritis. Organic foods are usually non-GMO, but you should look for the "non-GMO verified" stamp on the ingredients label when

you purchase products that include legumes and flour. To help you make organic choices, refer to the website of the Environmental Working Group (EWG) at www.ewg.org. There you can identify the foods with the highest pesticide levels—dubbed the "Dirty Dozen" by the nonprofit organization.

- Include healthy anti-inflammatory fats such as fish, flax, olive oil, avocados, coconut oil, nuts, and seeds.
- Choose grass-fed, pasture-raised, or free-range organic animals whenever possible. This will limit your exposure to the hormones, antibiotics, and pesticides that animals raised in typical feedlots eat. Also, the meat from grass-fed animals has higher quality, anti-inflammatory fats than meat from animals that are fed corn.
- Integrate liver-loving, gut-supporting, and antioxidant- and alkaline-producing food into your daily diet. Try to fill 70 percent of your plate at each meal with these foods:

Cruciferous Vegetables

- arugula
- bok choy
- broccoli
- broccoli rabe
- Brussels sprouts
- cabbage
- cauliflower
- Chinese cabbage (Napa cabbage)
- collard greens
- daikon (a type of radish)
- kale
- kohlrabi
- mustard greens
- radishes
- rutabaga
- turnips

Polyphenol-Rich Foods

Fruit

- apples
- apricots
- bananas
- all berries (especially dark-red and blue)
- grapefruit
- grapes
- lemons
- limes
- oranges
- peaches
- pears
- plums
- pomegranates

Vegetables

- artichokes
- okra
- red and green onions
- snap peas

Herbs and Spices

- cacao
- capers
- clove
- dill
- oregano
- parsley
- rosemary
- sage
- thyme

Beans

- black beans
- fava beans
- kidney beans
- pinto beans

Beverages
- black, red, and green tea
- fresh pressed juices

Nuts and Seeds
- cashews
- flaxseeds
- pecans
- pistachios
- walnuts

Antioxidant-Rich Dark, Leafy Greens
- collards
- kale
- lettuce: red leaf, green leaf, and romaine
- mustard greens
- spinach
- Swiss chard
- turnip greens

Prebiotic Foods for Your Gut
- asparagus
- cabbage
- chicory
- dandelion greens
- garlic
- Jerusalem artichokes
- leeks

Cultured and Fermented Food, for Probiotics
- Kimchi, sauerkraut, and other fermented vegetables (available in specialty or health food stores)
- Yogurt made from coconut or almonds

Foods to Eliminate

In these first two weeks of the Arthritis Protocol, you will focus on changing your diet by following an elimination diet. This is the best jump-start because many people have a dramatic improvement in how they feel just from eating differently. I want you to take these two weeks to settle into your new food plan before moving on to step 2's Two-Month Intensive Gut Repair. Ultimately, the goal of an elimination diet is to both help you feel better and identify which foods might be a problem for you so that you can create *your* personalized food plan when it's time for the Healthy Eating Plan in step 3, the Finish-What-You-Started Six-Month Program. The best way to determine if any of these foods are problematic is to eliminate them from your diet and then reintroduce them one at a time to see if you have a reaction.

Eliminate these foods:

- Processed food high in sugar, white flour, food dyes, and preservatives. These foods and chemicals promote the growth of the wrong kind of bacteria in your gut, and cause inflammation and oxidative stress in your body. Eating this way should be a permanent change. This includes fruit juices, high-sugar fruit, dried fruit, and all added sugar and artificial sweeteners except the herb stevia, the leaves of which are used as a noncaloric sweetener.
- Gluten, dairy, soy, corn, eggs, and peanuts. These foods are the most common triggers for digestive symptoms such as reflux, constipation, and abdominal discomfort, as well as other non-gut-related symptoms, including muscle and joint pain, headache, brain fog, and fatigue.
- Nightshade vegetables: tomatoes, potatoes, eggplant, and all peppers. These foods are commonly known to trigger joint pain.
- All alcohol and coffee.
- Fish with high levels of mercury such as tuna, swordfish, king mackerel, eel, and Chilean sea bass. See the list below, or you

can also go to the Environmental Working Group website (www
.ewg.org) for the most current recommendations.

Choosing Clean and Healthy Seafood

The following seafood is low in mercury and PCBs and high in healthy
omega-3 fats. In some cases, their origin has been noted to help you
know where they come from. Be careful: the same type of fish from
two different origins may have drastically different contamination
levels.

High-Omega 3s, Low-Mercury Fish

- anchovy (canned)
- Arctic char, farmed
- butterfish
- clams
- cod, Pacific, Atlantic
- crab (not blue)
- crayfish/crawfish
- flounder
- haddock (United States, Canada, Iceland, Norway)
- hake
- halibut, Pacific, moderate mercury, limit to three times per month
- herring, Atlantic (not Baltic or Chub)
- lobster
- mackerel, Atlantic (not king or Spanish)
- oysters, farmed
- pollock
- salmon (canned pink sockeye), wild Alaskan
- sardines
- scallops

- shrimp, pink, spot prawns
- sole
- trout (fresh water)
- tuna, skipjack, canned light (not solid white albacore), once a month
- whitefish, whiting

Worst Fish Choices

The list below contains seafood with the highest amount of mercury levels:

- bluefish
- Chilean sea bass
- eel
- grouper
- mackerel (king, Spanish, Gulf)
- marlin
- orange roughy
- red snapper
- rockfish/rock cod
- salmon, Atlantic farmed
- shark
- striped bass
- sturgeon
- swordfish
- tilefish
- tuna (albacore, yellowfin, Ahi, Bigeye, Bluefin, canned)
- wahoo

PROTEIN POWDERS

A protein shake for breakfast is a great option during an elimination diet because you can't eat many of your usual breakfast foods. Here are my tips for choosing protein powder:

- Choose a vegan powder such as pea, rice, or hemp protein, or a mix of these.
- Switch to a different powder every six months for a more ideal intake of different amino acids (the building blocks of proteins).
- Whey and soy should be avoided during the program.
- Choose a powder that has added benefits: for example, anti-inflammatory herbs, antioxidants, and L-glutamine for gut healing.

Your Leaky Gut Diet for Arthritis

This table summarizes your food plan for the next ten weeks, until after the Two-Month Intensive Gut Repair. There are plenty of foods to choose from, and you will not go hungry! Try to follow this as close to 100 percent as possible during this time. If you have to travel, attend a wedding or other event, or simply find yourself somewhere that makes it impossible to avoid restricted foods, then do your best and don't worry. The next day, just go back to your 100 percent focus on the program.

	FOOD TO INCLUDE	FOOD TO EXCLUDE
FRUIT	fresh or unsweetened frozen: apricots • berries (blackberries, blueberries, raspberries, strawberries) • cherries • grapefruit • kiwis • lemons and limes • melons • oranges • nectarines • tangerines	dried fruit • Remember to skip all fruit juice and dried versions of any fruit.

3-Step Arthritis Protocol and Guide

	FOOD TO INCLUDE	FOOD TO EXCLUDE
FRUIT (*cont.*)	peaches • persimmons • plums • pomegranates	
VEGETABLES	arugula • asparagus • avocado • bamboo shoots • beets • bok choy • broccoli • broccoli rabe • Brussels sprouts • cabbage (all types) • carrots • celeriac root • celery • cucumber • endive • fennel • greens (beets, chard, collard, chicory, dandelion, escarole, kale, mustard, purslane, radicchio) • green beans • horseradish • jicama • kohlrabi • leek • lettuce (all varieties) • mushrooms • okra • parsnips • peas (snap and snow only) • potatoes (sweet and yam) • radishes and daikon • sea vegetables (seaweed, kelp, nori, dulse, hiziki) • spinach • sprouts (all) • squash • turnips • watercress • water chestnuts	corn • eggplant • peppers (bell, cayenne, chili, paprika) • potatoes, white • tomatoes
GRAINS	gluten-free grains (quinoa, wild rice, millet, buckwheat, gluten-free oats)	products containing gluten (wheat, rye, barley, oats, spelt, kamut)
LEGUMES	adzuki beans • black beans • chickpeas • hummus • kidney beans • lentils • mung beans	soybean (including edamame, soy milk, soy sauce, tempeh, tofu)
NUTS	almonds • Brazil nuts • cashews • coconut (including coconut milk and flaked coconut) • hazelnuts and filberts • Macadamia nuts • pecans • pine nuts • pistachios • walnuts	peanuts (including peanut butter)

(*continued on next page*)

	FOOD TO INCLUDE	FOOD TO EXCLUDE
SEEDS	chia seeds • flaxseed • hemp seeds • pumpkin seeds • sesame seeds • sunflower seeds	
MEAT	beef • buffalo • elk • lamb • venison • wild game	all processed meat: canned meat • cold cuts (a thumbs-up, though, for products from Applegate Farms) • meat products in casing (frankfurters, sausages)
POULTRY	chicken (skinless) • Cornish hen • turkey	eggs
FISH Choose low-mercury fish. (See list on pages 200–201.)	anchovies • char (Arctic, farmed) • cod • halibut • herring • salmon (Alaskan) • sardines • Remember, you can have fish stocks of the above, if they do not contain excluded foods (MSG, gluten)	Skip smoked preparation of fish.
DAIRY PRODUCTS AND MILK SUBSTITUTES	unsweetened rice, almond, coconut, hemp, or other nondairy, nonsoy milk products	butter • cheese (all, including cottage cheese) • cream • kefir • milk (dairy) • nondairy creamers • frozen yogurt • ice cream • yogurt
FATS AND OILS	for cooking: avocado oil, coconut oil, ghee, grape seed oil • safflower (cold-pressed) oils • no heat or low-heat oils • olive oil (cold-pressed) • pumpkin seed oil	butter • margarine • mayonnaise • processed (hydrogenated) oils such as canola, vegetable, and spreads • processed (hydrogenated) spreads such as shortening
BEVERAGES	coffee or caffeinated tea (organic)—limit to one cup per day • seltzer or mineral water • tea (herbal, unsweetened) • water	alcoholic beverages • any prepared drink with sugar or artificial sweetener (soft drinks, sports drinks, bottled sweetened tea) • fruit juice • soda

	FOOD TO INCLUDE	FOOD TO EXCLUDE
HERBS, SPICES, AND CONDIMENTS	Spices: cardamom • cinnamon • clove • coriander • cumin • curry • ginger • nutmeg • turmeric All herbs, such as: basil • black pepper • bay leaves • chives • cilantro • dill • fennel • lemongrass • mint • oregano • parsley • rosemary • sage • iodized or pink Himalayan or real salt • tarragon • thyme Condiments: apple cider • balsamic vinegar • Dijon mustard • olives, black or green	chocolate • chutney • ketchup • mayonnaise • monosodium glutamate (MSG) • pepper (chili or cayenne) • relish • soy sauce, tamari, and teriyaki • salsa and sauces with a tomato or pepper base
SWEETENERS	honey • stevia (once per day and as little as possible)	agave • all artificial sweeteners (including aspartame and Splenda) • cane juice • evaporated high fructose • high-fructose corn syrup • molasses • sugar (white, raw, brown)

Arthritis Supplements

Oxidative stress is an imbalance that occurs when you don't have enough antioxidants to keep up with cell and tissue damage caused by free radicals. This is believed to contribute to the development of osteoarthritis and to fuel the inflammation and damage in autoimmune arthritis, too. In fact, many studies have shown high levels of oxidative stress in the joints of these patients, which suggests that antioxidants may be a very useful part of a therapeutic program.

I really believe that we should be able to get every necessary nutrient from the foods we eat because they usually contain a combination of various compounds that have their own health benefits—something you can't get from one isolated nutrient in a supplement. When you get your fill of antioxidants from all the colorful fruits and vegetables that grow abundantly in nature, you consume a broad range of vitamins. For example, an apple contains beta-carotene, vitamin C, and powerful antioxidant flavonoids such as epicatechin and quercetin, all coexisting in just one colorful food. Each one enhances the action of the other. That said, when you have a health condition that needs treatment with vitamins or antioxidants, it is often necessary to temporarily take a supplement as you would a medication in order to get higher doses of that nutrient.

I think of it as though I am writing a prescription. Good examples of this are the omega fatty acids such as fish oil (omega-3) and borage or evening primrose oil (omega-6). These are all powerful anti-inflammatory compounds found in foods like salmon and nuts, but they are often needed in concentrated amounts to reduce the pain and inflammation from all forms of arthritis. It is hard to get enough omega-3 every day from diet alone due to the increasing presence of heavy metals, polychlorinated biphenyls (PCBs), dioxins, and other environmental toxins in the fresh fish supply.

There are well over a thousand peer-reviewed studies on the benefits of taking omega-3 supplements. Beyond joint health, these include cardiovascular health, cognitive function, mood, immune function, inflammatory bowel disease, metabolic health, muscular strength and function, vision, and osteoporosis. Results have also shown that omega-3 supplements are best consumed in the triglyceride form (some supplements have it in a different chemical structure), which is how it is found naturally in food.[1] Multiple studies have shown the positive effects of fish oil supplementation on arthritis pain. In one study, when people with rheumatoid arthritis took 10 grams of cod liver oil every day, 39 percent of them significantly decreased their daily NSAID dosage and reported less pain.[2] Just note that when purchasing fish oil supplements, it is important to choose a brand that has clearly stated on its label that it is third-party tested for purity, potency, and freshness.

In a different clinical trial, RA patients took evening primrose oil, borage seed oil, or black currant seed oil (with the active ingredient GLA, an omega-6) for six months. Afterward, on a scale of 0 to 100, they rated their pain an average of 33 points lower than the study's control group, which received only a placebo. The people in the first group also showed greater improvement in their physical functioning.[3]

How do omegas work to improve inflammation and disease activity? It appears that in addition to their direct effect on producing anti-inflammatory compounds in the body, they also lower oxidative stress by boosting the activities of antioxidant enzymes. The most effective doses seem to be at least 2,500 milligrams of EPA and DHA, and 234 milligrams of GLA.[4]

Curcuminoids, which are natural polyphenols, are one of the strongest and most widely studied natural antioxidants and anti-inflammatories that you can get from food. They work by quenching lipid peroxidation, scavenging free radicals, and increasing the activity of antioxidant enzymes. They also suppress the formation of reactive oxygen species. Multiple studies have found that curcumin reduced pain and stiffness in people with osteoarthritis. For example, researchers at the University of Medical Sciences in Tehran, Iran, gave OA sufferers 1,500 milligrams per day of curcuminoids (combined with the active compound from pepper, piperine, to improve absorption). After six weeks they had an increase in two important blood markers for antioxidant activity. This study supports the idea that you should include curcumin both in your diet (in the form of the spice turmeric) and as a supplement. Based on other studies, my estimate is that the minimum effective dose is 500 milligrams per day of curcuminoids. At the beginning of the Arthritis Protocol, when a patient has a lot of inflammation and oxidative stress, I usually recommend 1,000 to 1,500 milligrams daily.[5]

In our discussion of both inflammatory arthritis and osteoarthritis, I mentioned the importance of oxidative stress and free radicals in fueling joint damage. Studies have found consistently that people with RA are deficient in vitamins C, D, B$_6$, B$_{12}$, and E, and minerals such as calcium, magnesium, zinc, and selenium.[6] Additional studies have also found deficits of specific antioxidants, like glutathione, and vitamins A, C, E, and beta-carotene.[7] To understand the importance of antioxidants, we need to look at whether using them therapeutically can improve arthritis symptoms. Researchers at Spain's University of Coruña found that giving the antioxidant resveratrol to mice increased antioxidant activity and reduced RA damage in joints.[8] In another study, from Taibah University in Medina, Saudi Arabia, having patients with rheumatoid arthritis add just 1 gram of vitamin C to their diets reduced all their RA markers and oxidative stress—as well as their symptoms.[9]

Given the research, and because we know that you are likely to have high oxidative stress as you begin your program, I recommend that you take the following antioxidant supplements each day in addition to enjoying the antioxidant-rich food on the Leaky Gut Diet for Arthritis:

- vitamin C: 1,000 milligrams
- vitamin E: 100 IU mixed tocopherols (the name of the compounds that collectively constitute vitamin E)
- vitamin A: 5,000 IU (as retinyl palmitate, the activated form of vitamin A)
- vitamin A: 5,000 IU (as beta-carotene)
- N-acetyl cysteine (also known as NAC, which raises glutathione): 300 to 600 milligrams
- lipoic acid: 200 to 400 milligrams
- curcumin: 1,000 milligrams
- resveratrol (optional): 100 to 200 milligrams

Here is the summary of all the supplement recommendations for the Arthritis Protocol:

- Omega-3 fish oil: 3 grams daily of EPA and DHA
- Omega-6: 500 milligrams daily of GLA from evening primrose or borage oil
- Soothe protein powder with antioxidants: one or two scoops in your daily morning shake
- vitamin D_3: 2,000 IU daily
- curcumin: 1,000 milligrams daily
- probiotics: 25 billion CFU daily
- multivitamin with antioxidants: two capsules daily
    - Mitocore dietary supplement, from Ortho Molecular Products; or a multivitamin with antioxidants, from Blum-HealthMD. Both include extra antioxidants, NAC, and lipoic acid
- vitamin C: 1,000 milligrams daily

It is easiest to take these bundled together so that you don't need to ingest so many pills. For example, the Blum multivitamin that I use includes A, C, and E, NAC, lipoic acid, and resveratrol; the Soothe protein shake contains curcumin and vitamins A, C, and E; the vitamin D that I use is a blend of vitamins A, D, E, and K; and I always offer a liquid omega option that includes EPA, DHA, and GLA, and can be added to a protein shake. See the following table for the exact program that I use for our arthritis patients at the Blum Center for Health, whether they have rheumatoid arthritis or osteoarthritis.

Supplement Instructions Using BlumHealthMD Products

	Breakfast	Dinner
fish oil capsules	2	2
GLA capsules	1	1
omega liquid (alternative to fish oil and GLA)	1 tablespoon	
multivitamin with antioxidants	2	
vitamin D_3	1	
curcumin	1	1
vitamin C	1	
Soothe protein powder	1–2 scoops	
probiotics	1	

Before leaving the topic of supplements, one last word about vitamin D. The idea that you can get the vitamin D you need from sunlight has been debunked, especially for most of the United States and European countries, where people live far from the equator. There are also no good food sources of vitamin D_3, which is the active form of vitamin D in humans, called cholecalciferol. Some vegetables, such as mushrooms, have D_2, called ergocalciferol, but it is hard for the body to convert it to D_3. I measure blood levels of vitamin D in all my patients, and out of the thousands of people we have seen at the Blum Center, I can count on one hand the number of them who maintained adequate vitamin D levels without taking a supplement. There is no perfect dose for everyone; it is based on the results of a blood test. The conventional range reported by the lab is that your vitamin D levels are normal if they fall between 30 and 100 nanograms per milliliter.

Lower levels than this have been linked to more severe symptoms and disease in people with RA and other arthritis conditions. Therefore, it is important to take vitamin D supplements to achieve normal levels.[10] This nutrient is critical for bone health, immune function, and treating autoimmunity, according to much research. My goal for my patients' vitamin D levels is narrower, between 50 and 60 nanograms per milliliter (ng/ml) of blood, and I find that most people start out between 25 and 35. I have patients begin with 4,000 to 5,000 IU daily; once repeat testing shows that they have reached the optimal range, I recommend a daily maintenance dose of 2,000 IU.

As you complete the Two-Week Jump-Start Leaky Gut Diet for Arthritis, you will begin the intensive work to repair your gut, and you should continue to take all of these new supplements and add what comes next.

Step 2: Two-Month Intensive Gut Repair

STEP 2: TWO-MONTH INTENSIVE GUT REPAIR AT-A-GLANCE SUMMARY

- *Continue* Leaky Gut Diet for Arthritis.
  - Elimination diet: remove gluten, dairy, soy, corn, eggs, peanuts, sugar, and processed flour products, alcohol, tomatoes, potatoes, eggplant, and peppers.

- *Continue* arthritis supplements.
  - omega-3 fish oil: 3 grams daily of EPA and DHA
  - omega-6: 500 milligrams daily of GLA from evening primrose or borage oil
  - Soothe protein powder with antioxidants: one or two scoops in your daily morning shake
  - vitamin D_3: 2,000 IU daily
  - curcumin: 1,000 milligrams daily

- probiotics: 25 billion CFU daily
- multivitamin with antioxidants: two capsules daily
- vitamin C: 1,000 milligrams daily

Add gut repair supplements.

- gut cleanse herbal blend: take one packet twice daily
- digestive enzymes: one or two with each meal
- probiotics: 25 billion CFU daily
- L-glutamine powder: one teaspoon twice daily

Suggested Schedule

Supplement	With Breakfast	With Dinner	Bedtime
fish oil capsules	2	2	
GLA capsules	1	1	
omega liquid (alternative to fish oil and GLA capsules)	1 tablespoon daily		
multivitamin with antioxidants	1–2		
vitamin D₃		1	
curcumin	1	1	
vitamin C	1		
Soothe protein powder	2 scoops		
probiotics			1
gut cleanse herbs (options listed on page 185)	1 packet of pills	1 packet of pills	
digestive enzymes (options listed on page 215)	1	1 with lunch and 1 with dinner	
glutamine powder	1 teaspoon	1 teaspoon	

Healing the gut is functional medicine 101. It is the first thing I learned in 2001 when I attended my first training course, Applying Functional Medicine in Clinical Practice, an experience that changed my life because it opened up a new medical world to me. I could see how to treat complex chronic inflammatory conditions by finding and treating the causes and triggers. Imagine, no more focusing on Band-Aid approaches that merely treat symptoms. This strategy could actually help heal people at the root of their problem. I felt awake, excited, and motivated to go out and practice this way.

The functional medicine approach to healing the gut has clear steps that guide the process. The first step is removing foods that might trigger gut or systemic inflammatory symptoms like joint pain, which you already started as part of the Leaky Gut Diet for Arthritis and you should continue while on this food plan. What comes next is removing harmful bacteria, yeast, and parasites; supporting digestion with enzymes; repairing the intestinal lining, which treats leaky gut; and using probiotics to restore good bacteria. This is how we will heal your gut and our focus in the Two-Month Intensive Gut Repair. Then you will move on to step 3, the Finish-What-You-Started Six-Month Program, to rebalance the gut so that these changes are permanent.

Based on these functional medicine steps for healing the gut, your supplement recommendations fall into four categories:

- herbs for treating dysbiosis
- enzymes for supporting digestion
- nutrients for healing leaky gut
- probiotics for restoring healthy gut bacteria

Herbs for Treating Dysbiosis

After learning the functional medicine basics and treating thousands of people for dysbiosis, I have crafted my own approach to this and created the Two-Month Intensive Gut Repair program. I have learned many things along the way. For example, while treating people with probiotics is a good place to start, and studies reveal some effectiveness, I always use herbs, and sometimes antibiotics or antiparasitic medication to treat dysbiosis. This enhances the effectiveness of probiotics to make a difference.

In my practice and in the Arthritis Protocol, we use a blend of different herbs to treat dysbiosis because bad bacteria and yeast in the gut are root triggers for inflammation in your joints. Here are my recommendations for treating dysbiosis. All herbs can be taken with meals or on an empty stomach—whatever your stomach likes best. Herbs such as oregano and thyme can irritate the stomach lining if you already have heartburn and take them when your stomach is empty. Remember, this list is offered as a suggestion; it is best to find different herb blends. You can take them as capsules, tablets, or tinctures, and when used in combination, the dosing might be lower than what I am recommending below. That is because, when added together, they have more power than when each one is used alone, and then you don't necessarily need the highest strength.

The herbs I suggest you take each day during your two months of treatment are listed below. Whichever blend you choose should be taken twice each day, just ten to fifteen minutes before breakfast and before dinner.

- berberine: 200 to 400 milligrams twice daily
- oregano oil: 100 to 200 milligrams twice daily
- thyme oil: 100 to 200 milligrams twice daily
- artemisia: 20 to 30 milligrams twice daily
- uva-ursi: 100 to 200 milligrams twice daily
- black walnut: 100 to 200 milligrams twice daily
- garlic: standardized to 5,000 micrograms allicin (the active ingredient in garlic) twice daily

The products that I use in my office include GI MicrobX, from Designs for Health; GI Synergy, from Apex Energetics; CandiBactin-BR, from Metagenics; Biocidin, from Bio Botanical Research; and

Gut Cleanse packets, from BlumHealthMD. (The packets also include enzymes and L-glutamine for an all-in-one option.)

Keep in mind that these herbs will begin to kill off the bad bacteria and yeast that you have in your digestive tract. As they die off, you might get a headache, feel more gas and bloating, and/or feel really tired—symptoms that should pass after a few days. However, if you're really uncomfortable, drop the dosage of the herbs or take a day off completely. These symptoms are a sign that you have lots of bad bacteria or yeast, and you might need to take it more slowly. Treating dysbiosis and improving the balance in your gut bacteria are absolutely crucial for your recovery from arthritis. Most people need two months for their initial gut cleanse program, and many need to repeat this treatment for another month within the first year. June is a good example of someone with severe RA who needed retreatment approximately every four to six months for two years. While I tend to use the Gut Cleanse packets most of the time, we also rotated and used the other products listed above. Again, for best results, I always use combination herbal formulas to treat dysbiosis, which is like using a broad-spectrum antibiotic to make sure all kinds of bacteria are affected by the treatment.

If you have heartburn or reflux, are taking antacids or proton pump inhibitors, or just feel like your stomach is irritated, it is a good idea to take a supplement to soothe your stomach at the same time you are treating your dysbiosis. I recommend taking these on an empty stomach to coat your stomach lining, which is usually easiest when you wake up and when you go to sleep. You can also take these nutrients at any time during the day that you have heartburn or reflux symptoms. All of these are good on their own, but, again, I often suggest a combination product that includes the following:

- L-glutamine powder: 3,000 milligrams one to three times daily. I suggest mixing one teaspoon of loose powder in water, which you can take with or without meals. This will also begin your treatment for leaky gut, so it serves two purposes.

- Dyglycerrated licorice (DGL): 500 to 1,000 milligrams three to four times daily. You can take chewables, loose powder, or capsule versions; just do so on an empty stomach or twenty minutes before meals.
- Slippery elm: 2 to 4 grams three times daily. Slippery elm comes in capsules or as a loose powder. Take on an empty stomach or twenty minutes before a meal.
- Aloe: look for aloe that has its laxative compounds removed, so that only the soothing qualities remain. It should say so on the label. Aloe comes in many forms: capsules, loose powder, and liquid.

My favorite products that blend the above are Glutagenics, from Metagenics; Heartburn Tx, from Vital Nutrients; GI-Revive, from Designs for Health; and Mend packets, from BlumHealthMD.

Enzymes for Supporting Digestion

If you have constipation, reflux, bloating after eating, or undigested food in your stool, you might need support for your digestion. Three organs in your body support proper digestion: the stomach, which makes acid; the pancreas, which makes enzymes; and the liver and the gall bladder, which secrete bile acids. All three are needed for good digestion and elimination, and a problem with any of them can be the cause of just about any and all digestive symptoms. Let's take a brief look at each of these, and then I will give you my recommendations for taking supplements.

First, let's talk about stomach acid, which, when taken as a supplement, is called betaine HCL (hydrochloric acid). There are many functions for your stomach acid, including sterilizing everything that you eat by killing the microbes that live in and on your food. It also suppresses the bad bacteria farther down in your intestines, which prevents SIBO, dysbiosis, and leaky gut. This is why antacids and proton pump inhibitors are on the list of medications that cause dysbiosis and leaky gut, and why you need to discontinue them if you want to treat it. If your stomach acid is low, you will have difficulty digesting and absorbing your food, be more likely to suffer acid reflux, have lower pancreatic enzyme activity, and be at a higher risk for developing an autoimmune disease and leaky gut. There is no easy test for low stomach acid; the simplest strategy that I use if I want to add betaine to a treatment plan is to include it as an ingredient in a complete digestive enzyme supplement.

Your liver makes bile acids, which are stored in your gall bladder. When your stomach and the upper part of your small intestine sense fat in your meal, the gall bladder pumps out the bile. If you feel you need more help with fat digestion even after taking a basic digestive enzyme (see below), you might want to find a more complete digestion support formula that includes ox bile. (This will be on the ingredient list on the bottle.) One example is Ortho Digestzyme by Ortho Molecular. You can also enhance your bile flow by taking taurine and dandelion, either separately or together.

The pancreas manufactures digestive enzymes and then releases them into the bloodstream in response to sensors that detect food and an acid environment. Enzymes are important for helping your digestive tract break down food into the smallest particles, which reduces your risk of food sensitivities because the tiny food particles can evade the immune system. And enzymes help you digest and absorb nutrients better. For step 2, the Two-Month Intensive Gut Repair, I recommend taking a digestive enzyme supplement with every meal. Look for one that includes any mixture of the ingredients named below. Start with one type; you might need to try a few, though, until you find the right blend that improves your symptoms. Take the enzyme at the beginning of each meal. If, after two weeks, you don't notice any change in your symptoms, try taking two with each meal.

- Pancreatin (a mixture of the digestive enzymes lipase, amylase, and protease; animal derived): 800 to 24,000 USP (United States Pharmacopoeia) lipase activity (the standard used to measure the strength of the enzyme activity). This formula is the most potent and usually my first choice unless you are a vegetarian or simply prefer the vegetarian enzymes.

- Vegetarian enzymes blend amylase, protease, lipase, bromelain, papain, and other enzymes for digesting carbohydrates, such as maltase, lactase, and cellulase. They are often aspergillus derived, so if you are allergic to mold, you might need to take pancreatin.
- Bromelain contains mainly proteases for digesting protein: 1,200 to 2,400 milk clotting units (MCU); 250 to 500 milligrams taken with meals.
- Papain, from papaya, contains mainly proteases for digesting protein; 50,000 USP; 100 to 200 milligrams taken with meals.
- When choosing bile acids, find a digestive enzyme blend that includes ox bile: 500 to 1,000 milligrams with food.
- Taurine helps you make better bile and improves bile flow: 500 to 1,000 milligrams with meals.
- Dandelion root also helps you make better bile and improves bile flow: 2 to 4 grams three times daily with meals; or 5 milliliters of 1:1 fluid extract (a liquid preparation containing alcohol as a solvent) three times daily with meals.
- Betaine: 150 to 250 milligrams per capsule. Take one or two with meals, or look for it as an ingredient in a digestive enzyme formula.
- To help stimulate your own stomach acid production, choose one to try at a time:
  - Ginger: 500 milligrams to 2 grams before meals
  - Gentian: 1 to 2 milliliters. 1:5 tincture before meals. A tincture is a medicine dissolved in alcohol, and the 1:5 is a measure of the strength of the tincture
  - Swedish bitters: 1 to 2 milliliters before meals
- Suggested products, choose one:
  - Basic pancreatic enzymes, vegan formula: Vital Zymes Complete, from Klaire Labs; Digestzyme-V, from Ortho

Molecular; Plant Enzyme Digestive Formula, from Designs for Health; Enzyme Support, from BlumHealthMD.

- Complete digestion formulas for anyone who has had his or her gallbladder removed or who needs extra power digesting fat: Ortho Digestzyme, from Ortho Molecular; Complete Digestion Support, from BlumHealthMD.
- Gut Cleanse packets, from BlumHealthMD: if you choose these packets to provide the herbs for your Intensive Gut Repair, you will not need to purchase separate enzymes because they have one plant enzyme capsule in each packet.

Nutrients for Healing Leaky Gut

It takes time to heal the intestinal lining, so I recommend taking these supplements as soon as you begin your Two-Month Intensive Gut Repair and stay on them through the Finish-What-You-Started Six-Month Program. The most popular and well-studied supplement for treating leaky gut is L-glutamine, which we talked about in chapter 6, "How to Heal the Gut." Glutamine comes in capsules or powders, and I often recommend powders to get the higher dosing that is necessary for those with arthritis.

Here are the supplements you should take:

- L-glutamine powder: 3,000 to 4,000 milligrams twice daily. Just mix one teaspoon with water or add to your breakfast smoothie
- Curcumin: 500 milligrams twice daily
- Zinc carnosine: 75 milligrams once daily
  - As an option, take 30 milligrams of zinc daily as part of your vitamin regimen
- Suggested products:
  - L-glutamine, from Designs for Health; Glutagenics, from Metagenics; Strengthen powder, from BlumHealthMD

- Curcumin: Meriva 500, from Thorne; Curcu-Evail, from Designs for Health; CurcuPlex, from Xymogen; curcumin, from BlumHealthMD
- Zinc carnosine: Zinlori, from Metagenics; zinc carnosine, from Integrative Therapeutics. Also found in blends such as Heartburn Tx, from Vital Nutrients; GI-Revive, from Designs for Health; Mend packets, from BlumHealthMD

TWO-MONTH INTENSIVE GUT REPAIR PROGRAM USED AT THE BLUM CENTER FOR HEALTH, WITH SPECIFIC SUPPLEMENTS FROM BLUMHEALTHMD:

INSTRUCTIONS

1. Gut Cleanse packets: two boxes with sixty packets each. This is an herbal, antibacterial, and antiyeast formula that also has some anti-parasitic activity. Take this twice a day, in the morning and evening, ten to fifteen minutes before meals. This is the core part of your treatment, and two boxes will last you sixty days.
    a. First and second day: take one packet in the morning only, ten to fifteen minutes before breakfast.
    b. Beginning day three: take one packet twice daily—the first packet ten to fifteen minutes before breakfast; the second, ten to fifteen minutes before dinner. Take all the packets in the box.
    c. Keep in mind that if you have lots of bad bacteria or yeast (moderate to severe dysbiosis), you might have what's called a die-off reaction. This means that as the bad microbes are killed with the Gut Cleanse supplements, you might feel more fatigue, brain fog, and possibly a headache or GI symptoms such as nausea. If the side effects are uncomfortable, cut back the dose to one packet daily for a day or two, and then go up again to the full dose. That said, you might not experience any side effects at all.
    d. You should notice a reduction in digestion and gut-related symptoms (if you have any) by the end of the first week, especially if

you are following the Leaky Gut Diet for Arthritis (as you should be!). However, for some people, this can take longer.

    e. Each packet contains two capsules of herbs (berberine, barberry, magnesium caprylate, tribulus extract, uva-ursi, artemisinin, black walnut (hull) extract, two capsules of oregano, one capsule of L-glutamine, one capsule of vegetarian digestive enzymes.

2. Probiotics: choose a multistrain formula of at least 25 billion CFU.

    a. We recommend taking one capsule at bedtime during your two months of treatment because you should not take probiotics the same time of day that you take your Gut Cleanse packets. Once you move on to step 3, the Finish-What-You-Started Six-Month Program, you can take your probiotic with any meal during the day.

3. Soothe protein powder with antioxidants for gut integrity: one canister of protein powder has twenty-eight scoops of powder and makes a delicious and filling breakfast protein shake.

    a. Use one to two scoops of powder each day. Mix with water, juice, or almond, rice, or coconut milk, or put in a blender and add your favorite fruit. We have several smoothie recipes for you to try in this book and also in my first book, *The Immune System Recovery Plan*.

    b. Stay on this shake for the full two-month Intensive Gut Repair program. If you like this protein shake, you can continue it as long as you like. In fact, it is a terrific option to have this breakfast shake for the next step, the Finish-What-You-Started Six-Month Program.

4. Strengthen powder: concentrated L-glutamine for enhanced treatment of leaky gut.

    a. Add one teaspoon of Strengthen powder to your shake every morning and have another teaspoon mixed in plain water ten to fifteen minutes before dinner when you take your second daily Gut Cleanse packet.

Probiotics for Restoring Healthy Gut Bacteria

The final part of your Intensive Gut Repair is to begin the process of restoring the good bacteria with probiotics. As I've mentioned, probiotics are the beneficial bacteria, and prebiotic foods are the "fertilizer" to help them grow. Both are critical for repairing the intestinal lining, and you will be getting plenty of prebiotics in your new food plan, which is why I don't usually prescribe a separate prebiotic supplement.

As you learned in chapter 6, "How to Heal the Gut," the bacterial strains with the most powerful anti-inflammatory effects in arthritis are *Lactobacilli*: *L. casei, L. acidophilus, L. reuteri, L. rhamnosus GG*, and *L. salivarius*. There is also convincing evidence of benefits from *Bifidobacterium bifidum. Bifidobacterium infantis, E. coli* Nissle, and *Lactobacillus plantarum* were found to improve tight junctions and heal leaky gut, even if they weren't studied for their effects specifically on arthritis. Therefore, for probiotics, I recommend a combination formula with as many of these strains as possible. For the Two-Month Intensive Gut Repair, I recommend taking a probiotic daily. But while you are treating your dysbiosis with herbs, take the probiotic at bedtime because you should not take the probiotic within two hours of the herbs. Look for one that includes any mixture of the following ingredients, and with a total of 25 billion to 50 billion live organisms. You can take this as a capsule, tablet, or loose powder mixed in food or any beverage.

Here are the probiotics I recommend:

Lactobacillus Species

- *Lactobacillus casei*
- *Lactobacillus acidophilus*
- *Lactobacillus reuteri*
- *Lactobacillus rhamnosus*
- *Lactobacillus salivarius*
- *Lactobacillus plantarum*
- *Lactobacillus bulgaricus*
- *Lactobacillus paracasei*

Bifidobacterium Species

- *Bifidobacterium bifidum*
- *Bifidobacterium longum*
- *Bifidobacterium lactis*
- *Bifidobacterium breve*

Saccharomyces Species

- *Saccharomyces boulardii*: 200 to 500 milligrams daily. This good yeast is especially useful for protecting your gut bacteria when you take antibiotics, and for preventing and treating *Candida* (yeast) overgrowth.

Suggested products: Ther-Biotic Complete, from Klaire Labs; Probiotics, from BlumHealthMD.

Oral Dysbiosis Program for Rheumatoid Arthritis

As part of the Two-Month Intensive Gut Repair, some of you will need to treat your oral microbiome, which are the bacteria in your mouth, because there are many studies (reviewed in chapter 1, "Rheumatoid Arthritis") showing that this is an important issue for people with inflammatory arthritis—especially rheumatoid arthritis (and early or seronegative RA)—and is linked to joint inflammation. Therefore, if you have RA, you will need to treat this at the same time you are treating your gut. To do this, go to a holistic dentist or periodontist (a specialist in gum disease) to be evaluated and treated for gingivitis. Even if the periodontist tells you that your gums are okay, I still suggest that you follow the oral dysbiosis program I recommend.

If you have any other inflammatory arthritis condition, such as psoriatic arthritis or ankylosing spondylitis, you should get checked by your dentist too, especially if you have any of these symptoms of periodontal disease: gums that are red, inflamed, and sore, or that bleed easily when flossing. Your dentist can refer you to a periodontist for evaluation and treatment. If you discover that you do have inflammation in your gums, then you should follow the program for treating oral dysbiosis that I will share here. If you have osteoarthritis, the good news is that you can skip this section and just focus on your gut for step 2.

I send all of my RA patients to the holistic dentist or periodontist for an evaluation of their gums, or gingiva. If needed, they are encouraged to treat gingivitis with conventional approaches. At the same time, I prescribe an oral health program that is done daily during the same two months as the gut treatment program. (After that, I suggest doing it one to three times per week to maintain good oral hygiene.) The program is very simple and is done when you wake up and go to sleep. You can use a Waterpik machine (available at drugstores, mass merchandisers, or online) twice a day and add an antibacterial formula in the water that can help cleanse the gums and remove plaque. Or you can use a mouth rinse where you swish and then spit out the herbal treatment.

Recommended Products

- For the mouth rinse: Herb Pharm Oral Health Tonic Herbal Mouthwash. Put one dropperful in two ounces of water, swish for sixty seconds, and then spit out, twice daily.
- For the Waterpik: Nature's Answer PerioBrite Cleanse Oral Cleansing Concentrate. Put two pumpfuls in the water reservoir, twice daily.

Step 3: Finish-What-You-Started Six-Month Program

STEP 3: FINISH-WHAT-YOU-STARTED SIX-MONTH PROGRAM AT-A-GLANCE SUMMARY

NUTRITION
- *Stop* Leaky Gut Diet for Arthritis.
- *Begin* Healthy Eating Plan.

SUPPLEMENTS

- *Continue* arthritis supplements:
  - omega-3 fish oil: 3 grams daily of EPA and DHA
  - omega-6: 500 milligrams daily of GLA from evening primrose or borage oil
  - vitamin D$_3$: 2,000 IU daily
  - curcumin: 500 milligrams daily (new dose)
  - multivitamin with antioxidants: two capsules daily
  - vitamin C: 1,000 milligrams daily (optional)
- *Continue* gut repair supplements:
  - digestive enzymes: one or two with each meal
  - probiotics: 50 billion CFU daily (new dose)
  - L-glutamine powder: one teaspoon once daily (new dose)
- *Add* joint support:
  - undenatured type 2 collagen: 10 milligrams daily

Mind-Body Practice for Treating Trauma and Stress

- *Begin* daily mind-body exercise for relaxation and self-awareness.

Suggested Schedule

Supplement	With Breakfast	With Dinner
fish oil capsules	2	2
GLA capsules	1	1
omega liquid (alternative to fish oil and GLA capsules)	1 tablespoon daily	
multivitamin with antioxidants	2	
vitamin D$_3$		1
curcumin	1	1
vitamin C	1	

(continued on next page)

Supplement	With Breakfast	With Dinner
Soothe protein powder	1–2 scoops	
probiotics	1	1
digestive enzymes	1	1 with lunch and 1 with dinner
L-glutamine powder	1 teaspoon	
undenatured type 2 collagen 10 milligram	1	

Creating Resiliency

Shifting your body on the deepest level toward resiliency and vibrant health is the ultimate goal of the Arthritis Protocol. This is what I call shifting your terrain. If you just follow the diet and gut cleanse part of this program, you will feel better. That said, the effect will be short lived if you go back to your old habits when you finish. Additionally, if you don't try to understand how stress and trauma influence your health, it may prevent the terrain shift needed for permanent healing in your body. The truth is that healing the gut takes time and commitment, as you've seen from the patients' stories I've shared, so it is important to release any expectations. This way, you won't be concerned or worried when it seems to be taking months, or longer, to heal completely.

In 2001 I took my first functional medicine training and was very excited at the prospect that I now had the tools to help people feel better quickly. And in the early years of my practice, it was a very euphoric experience to observe the powerful changes that happened in people's lives when they followed the first months of the functional medicine detox or gut healing program. It was like the honeymoon after the wedding! It was incredible and a joy for me to witness after years of practicing conventional medicine and my increasing despair over the approach to people with complex, chronic illness, which merely tries to control their symptoms.

Yet after the euphoria came the hard reality (like settling into a long marriage after the honeymoon!). Quick fixes are a great jump-start, but they are only a beginning; they don't permanently *fix* any-thing. For deeper, long-lasting change, and the possibility of an actual cure of your symptoms and illness, you need to *finish what you started* after the jump-start and maintain it with a program that becomes a permanent change in your lifestyle.

I learned how to help my patients finish what they started after many years of figuring out what comes after the honeymoon. Working with my autoimmune and arthritis patients, it became very clear that restoring healthy gut bacteria and repairing the intestinal lining were at the heart of what needed to be accomplished, and I discovered that while you will definitely feel better, complete healing doesn't happen within the first few months of treatment for most people. It is a pro-cess that needs to continue with a program that isn't as intense but maintains important basic principles of nutrition, mindfulness, and gut support.

Everyone is different, and how long this takes depends on the severity of your disease and symptoms. For newly diagnosed rheu-matoid arthritis with mild symptoms and low antibody levels, it will probably take under a year; for someone who has been on medica-tion for many years, with high antibody titers and lots of symptoms, it will take longer. The Finish-What-You-Started Six-Month Program is meant to be the beginning of a lifestyle program that you adopt as your long-term healthy home base, with guiding principles that will continue to heal your body from the inside out. The length of time until your symptoms are gone also depends on how closely you follow the program. This is well illustrated with my patient Sherry. While she was certainly happy and feeling much better, it took almost three years for her to heal completely because she didn't follow the program exactly as I had recommended. My point is that there are many ways to get there, which is why I offer a variety of patients' stories through-out this book.

Keep in mind that the goal of the entire 3-Step Arthritis Protocol is not only a complete cure of your arthritis pain but also to create a deeper resiliency within you so that if you go on vacation, are exposed to an infection, or have a period of intense or traumatic stress, you won't have a relapse or flare-up of your symptoms. *Not having a relapse is really the ultimate measure of success, and to do that, we have to build resiliency. Nothing replaces time for this to happen.* Over time, following the Healthy Eating Plan and having a daily mindfulness practice of some kind, you will begin to become bulletproof to what life throws your way. Your diet and the stress that comes into your body are the two most influential factors in your gut health, so if we really want to repair your gut, which is the gateway to stopping your inflammation and pain, you must follow these changes long term.

I want to share two stories of resiliency to illustrate this point. Recently, I traveled to Mexico City to attend the funeral mass of our dear friend who died too young from prostate cancer. It had been a year since my diagnosis of episcleritis and arthritis, and well over eight months since I'd had my last symptom flare-up, which happened after a vacation where I splurged on just about everything. The day after the mass, we spent time with our friend's widow, who took me and my husband, Bruce, to an up-and-coming neighborhood for lunch and to stroll around.

As we were walking along one of the side streets, a man jumped in front of us with a gun. It took us all a few seconds to realize what was happening. My husband threw his wallet and phone at the guy, who grabbed them and ran away. As you can imagine, we were all very shaken up and traumatized.

For the next twenty-four hours until our flight home, we didn't leave our hotel. At the airport, just being in a crowd where many of the men looked like the guy who robbed us gave me flashbacks of this horrible incident. I didn't feel safe and could sense the hypervigilance of my nervous system through a racing heart all the way home. All the while, I told myself that I had better do something to release this trauma, or my arthritis would come back. We finally got home, and the next day, I tried to meditate but discovered that I felt too unsettled in my body to sit quietly. Thank goodness I had the tools to help myself recover because of what I have learned at the Center for Mind-Body Medicine. I started a daily practice of shaking and dancing, also called dynamic meditation, and slowly felt my nervous system come back into balance. (I will share the resources for how to learn this exercise later in the chapter.) Within a week, I no longer had memories and thoughts that triggered a stress response in my body. And the best news is that I did not have a flare-up of my eye and joint symptoms.

I think there are two take-home messages in my story. The first is that I had developed a deep resilience in my body that helped prevent me from getting sick again. This resiliency had developed because I had stuck with my recovery program for one year and counting, including the Healthy Eating Plan and daily meditation. The second message is that when something happens and you find yourself in dangerous waters, off the wagon with food or experiencing severe stress of any kind, *you must do whatever you can to get yourself back on track as soon as possible* so that these negative outside forces don't cause internal damage that can lead to a relapse. Because I have good self-care tools in my tool box and I recognized that I needed them, I was able to stay healthy through something very traumatizing.

Finally, one more story of resiliency and another example of this. One weekend I attended a conference and was able to relax and hang out with many of my functional medicine colleagues. It turned out that two of my friends experienced significant exposure to mold in the past year. One told me that she was very sick for three months, and because she also had the stress of writing a new book, it was all too much and overwhelmed her body. She was still trying to recover from her fatigue and digestive issues when I saw her. Another colleague told me that she had to move out of her house because of mold. While it was a terrible and stressful experience, she kept up her Healthy Eating Plan, her twice-daily meditation practice, and her daily exercise regimen. As a result, neither the mold nor the stress got to her, and she didn't get sick. (Those were her words, not mine.) She was proud that her self-care had created resiliency in her system so that she could weather this storm so well.

This highlights perfectly the idea of resiliency and the concept of terrain. Her terrain was in great shape because of her self-care practices, and this had created resiliency in her body, like a bulletproof vest that protected her from a potentially harmful exposure. The goal of step 3, the Finish-What-You-Started Six-Month Program, is for you to start building your bulletproof vest, so that you will have protection as you travel through the inevitable ups and downs of life. During this terrain-shifting, deeper-healing phase, you will focus on the following:

- Transitioning out of the Leaky Gut Diet for Arthritis and into the Healthy Eating Plan, a basic anti-inflammatory, gut-supportive food plan
- Learning, through trial and error, which core supplements are most effective for reducing inflammation and supporting your gut
- Exploring how your mind and spirit affect your health and learning tools to bring balance to this system
- Talking to your doctor about whether you can lower the dosage of your medication(s)

Reintroducing Foods

As you move on to the Finish-What-You-Started Six-Month Program, you will first transition out of the elimination diet. It is time to reintroduce all the foods you have been avoiding: gluten, dairy, soy, corn, eggs, tomatoes, potatoes, eggplant, peppers, peanuts, alcohol, and coffee. This is a very important step, and it is essential that you add back one food at a time and record your reactions, so that you can identify the foods to which you are sensitive. They can be added back in any order, but it is best to start with eggs, and then soy, and then corn because these three foods are in other foods. Even if you don't have a noticeable reaction to gluten or dairy, I still recommend avoiding them for the next six months on the Healthy Eating Plan.

Here are your instructions:

- Introduce one food at a time. Eat that food several times over two days. Observe on day three. If no reaction, add the next food on day four.
- If you do have a reaction, such as headache, rash, brain fog, fatigue, digestive reaction, or any other symptom, write it down in a food journal or a place you keep notes on your phone so that you don't forget. Once you know that a particular food isn't good for you, remove it again and wait for the reaction to go away before reintroducing the next eliminated food. Usually this takes only a day or two.
- As you continue with the Healthy Eating Plan, you need to avoid foods that triggered a reaction. These are your food sensitivities. Some of you might be okay using the 90 percent rule: 90 percent of the time, don't eat the food; 10 percent of the time, you can eat it, which is about one or two times a week. Others, however, will need to be more vigilant and eliminate the food completely. It depends on how severe your reaction was and how sick you felt.
- Every three to six months, try eating the foods that you are sensitive to and see if you still have a reaction. As you continue to deepen your healing and improve your gut terrain, you will be able to eat them—but in small amounts, and not every day.
- Although I encourage you to continue limiting gluten and dairy, you can try small amounts of grass-fed organic butter and goat-milk or sheep-milk dairy products such as full-fat yogurt. If you don't experience a reaction, you can eat them two or three times each week.

The Healthy Eating Plan

Now you are ready for the Healthy Eating Plan, created to be a sane, easy-to-follow approach to nutrition that you can adopt as a lifelong way of eating. Elimination diets and overly restrictive diets are not sustainable; you need something you can live with and that you are not stressed about. Your goal is to follow these guidelines 90 percent of the time, so that these foods work their way deeper into your cells to treat oxidative stress and provide fiber and nutrients to permanently shift your gut flora into a robust and anti-inflammatory microbiome. This plan teaches you the foods to emphasize and the ones to minimize. It is not a weight loss plan, but if, say, you have osteoarthritis and are overweight, it will definitely help you lose the body fat that might be driving some of your inflammation.

The food plan has five simple goals:

1. **Focus on Eating Foods That Reduce Inflammation**. This includes colorful, antioxidant-rich produce; healthy fats, such as nuts, seeds, and avocados; low-mercury fish such as sardines and wild Alaskan king salmon; and olive oil and other foods that add an alkaline boost to the body when they are metabolized. It also includes herbs such as turmeric, ginger, and rosemary.

2. **Include Foods That Support Gut Health**. These include all the foods I mentioned in the section called "Diet and Gut Health" on page 144 and the foods to emphasize in the chart on page 234.

3. **Avoid Inflammatory Foods 90 Percent of the Time**. It is not sustainable to try to be perfect 100 percent of the time. Avoid foods that you are sensitive to for six months, as well as processed sugar and flour products such as white breads, cookies, and cakes—even if they say "gluten free." Limit dairy products, beef that is not grass fed and organic, and acid-producing food. The rule of thumb is that a meal should consist of 70 percent alkaline-producing foods and 30 percent acid-producing foods. In general, all protein produces acid because of how it is metabolized, but animal proteins increase acid in the body more than vegetable proteins such as legumes do. Try to increase your

vegetarian protein, and, in either case, fill your plate with vegetables so that the protein and grains represent only 30 percent of the meal. Limit the worst acid producers (listed below), although bear in mind that it is okay to eat these foods in moderation as part of a balanced approach to eating.

HIGHEST ACID-PRODUCING FOODS: LIMIT TO 30 PERCENT OF YOUR DIET

- all animal protein: beef, chicken, turkey, pork, lamb, fish, shellfish
- all dairy (except ghee)
- legumes (except lentils, which are alkaline)
- tomatoes
- walnuts, Brazil nuts, pistachios, hazelnuts
- coffee (tea is alkaline)
- alcohol, especially beer
- soda and sugared drinks
- cocoa
- all grains except quinoa. The more processed the flour, the higher the acid.
- sulfur-covered dried fruit

4. **Avoid Toxins**. The antioxidants and greens you will be eating help your body excrete heavy metals such as mercury, along with pesticides and plastic residues. While these toxins are all around us, you can and must take steps to reduce your exposures, and this is what I call living a low-toxin lifestyle. Drink alcohol in moderation—about one or two drinks a week—and eat organic when possible. (Look at the "Dirty Dozen" and the "Clean Fifteen"—the foods that you don't need to buy organic, like avocado, pineapple, cabbage, onion, and asparagus—on the

Environmental Working Group website at www.ewg.org, and follow the low-mercury-fish list on page 200.)

5. **Follow Dr. Blum's Five Guiding Principles for Choosing Food**:

    a. Reduce refined sugar, high-fructose corn syrup, and refined grains. Minimize and eat these only once a week as a treat, occasionally twice.

    b. Improve the quality of the fats you eat by removing refined oils and hydrogenated fat. Make a permanent change in what you use for cooking and salad dressings.

    c. Improve the quality of animal protein by choosing organic grass-fed and finished beef, free-range chicken, and sustainably farmed, low-mercury fish 90 percent of the time. Focus on changing what you buy and cook for yourself and your family at home. Then you can be less vigilant when you eat out.

    d. Increase fiber, micronutrients, and phytonutrients with more vegetables and fruits, and choose organic when possible. Remember, aim for filling 70 percent of your plate at each meal with vegetables.

    e. Limit salt, food dyes, and preservatives. (This happens naturally when you limit processed foods.) Plan ahead, do your grocery shopping on the weekends, and cook and freeze food and soups so that you aren't relying on fast food or processed packages for your meals.

THE HEALTHY EATING PLAN FOOD LIST

Category	Food to Emphasize	Food to Minimize (Avoid 90 Percent of the Time)
Fruit Choose deeply colored, in season, organic, and locally grown.	avocados all fresh or unsweetened frozen fruits, unless otherwise indicated	juices and dried fruit (too sweet)

Category	Food to Emphasize	Food to Minimize (Avoid 90 Percent of the Time)
Nonstarchy Vegetables Choose deeply colored, in season, organic, and locally grown.	all fresh, raw, steamed, fermented, sautéed, juiced, or roasted vegetables	You might need to continue to limit the nightshades: tomatoes, white potatoes, eggplants, bell peppers, paprika, salsa, chili peppers, cayenne, chili powder.
Starchy Vegetables	beets, butternut squash, carrots, parsnips, potatoes, non-GMO organic corn.	
Fermented Foods (Gut Friendly)	kimchi, sauerkraut, kefir, tempeh, pickled food, natto (fermented soybeans).	
Prebiotic Foods (Gut Friendly)	asparagus, cabbage, chicory, garlic, leeks, Jerusalem artichokes, inulins, raw dandelion greens, onions.	
Grains	quinoa, buckwheat, millet, amaranth, rice.	gluten-containing grains: wheat, rye, spelt, kamut.
Legumes	adzuki, black, garbanzo (chickpeas), kidney, and mung beans; lentils, peas, non-GMO organic soy foods such as edamame, tofu, and tempeh.	
Nuts and Seeds	nuts and seeds and their butters, with no added sugar or oils.	
Meat and Fish (Protein) Choose low-mercury fish; 100 percent grass-fed and finished organic meats, organic poultry	all canned (water-packed), frozen, or fresh, low-mercury fish; chicken, turkey, eggs, beef, wild game, shellfish, lamb.	frankfurters, canned meats, cold cuts (unless from Applegate Farms), sausage.
Dairy Products and Milk Substitutes Choose unsweetened.	Milk substitutes such as almond, coconut, hemp, rice; small amounts of grass-fed organic butter, and goat-milk or sheep-milk dairy products.	Products from cow's milk such as cheese, cottage cheese, cream, frozen yogurt, ice cream, yogurt, "nondairy" creamers.

(continued on next page)

Category	Food to Emphasize	Food to Minimize (Avoid 90 Percent of the Time)
Fats and Oils	For cooking: avocado, coconut, grapeseed, macadamia oils and ghee; low-heat, no-heat: flax, olive, pumpkin, sesame oils.	margarine, mayonnaise, shortening, processed (hydrogenated) oils such as canola, vegetable; spreads.
Beverages Choose unsweetened.	filtered or distilled water, all teas, seltzer, and mineral water; organic coffee (one cup per day).	Minimize alcoholic beverages; avoid soda/soft drinks.
Herbs, Spices, and Condiments	All spices unless otherwise indicated. For example, use carob, chocolate, cinnamon, cumin, dill, garlic, ginger, oregano, parsley, rosemary, tarragon, thyme, turmeric. Mustard (without artificial ingredients). Vinegar.	High-sugar chutneys, MSG, relish, and other store-bought condiments with unknown ingredients.
Sweeteners	Small amounts of honey, maple syrup, stevia.	agave, artificial sweeteners such as aspartame and Splenda; sugar, brown sugar, corn syrup, evaporated cane juice, high-fructose corn syrup.

Grocery Shopping List

Vegetables
arugula
artichokes
asparagus
bamboo shoots
bok choy
broccoli, broccoli rabe
Brussels sprouts
cabbage (all types)
carrots

cauliflower

celeriac root

celery

chard/Swiss chard

chives

cilantro

cucumber

eggplant

endive

fennel

garlic

greens (beet, collard, chicory, dandelion, escarole, kale, mustard, purslane, radicchio, turnip)

green beans

horseradish

jicama

kohlrabi

leeks

lettuce, all varieties

mushrooms

microgreens

okra

onions

parsley

peppers (all)

radishes, daikons

scallions, shallots

sea vegetables (seaweed, kelp, nori, dulse, hiziki)

snap peas/snow peas

sprouts (all)

spinach

squash (delicate, pumpkin, spaghetti, yellow, zucchini)

tomatoes

watercress

Vegetables (Starchy)
acorn squash
beets
butternut squash
plantains
potatoes (purple, red, sweet, yellow)
root vegetables (parsnips, rutabagas)
yams

Fruit
apples
apricots (fresh)
bananas
blackberries
blueberries
cherries
grapefruit
grapes
kiwis
melons (all)
nectarines
oranges
papayas
peaches
pears
persimmons
plums
prunes
tangerines

Dairy Products and Milk Substitutes
yogurt and kefir: coconut or almond milk
milk: almond, coconut, hazelnut, hemp (unsweetened)

Meat and Fish
fish (omega-3 rich): cod, sardines, Alaskan salmon, halibut, herring, shrimp
meat: beef, buffalo, elk, lamb, venison, other wild game
poultry: chicken, Cornish hen, turkey
eggs

Gluten-Free Grains
amaranth
brown rice
millet
quinoa
wild rice

Fats and Oils
minimally refined, cold-pressed, organic, non-GMO preferred
avocados
coconut milk, light (canned)
coconut milk, regular (canned)
olives, black or green

Oils for Cooking
avocado
coconut
ghee (clarified butter)
olive oil (cold pressed)

Salad Oils
avocado
flaxseed
hemp seed
olive (extra-virgin)
pumpkin seed
sesame

sunflower

walnut

Nuts and Seeds

Nuts

almonds

Brazil nuts

cashews

coconut flakes (unsweetened)

hazelnuts

pecan halves

pine nuts

pistachios

walnut halves

Seeds

chia seeds

hemp seeds

flaxseed (ground)

pumpkin seeds

sesame seeds

sunflower seeds

All of the above can be consumed as nut butters and spreads (for example, tahini).

Legumes

adzuki

all beans and bean soups

edamame

hummus

lentils (brown, green, red)

mung beans

split peas (yellow, green—cooked)

All the above beans can be bought dried or canned (BPA free), without added sugar.

Beverages
coffee
herbal tea (noncaffeinated)
distilled water
mineral, sparkling water
spring water

Herbs, Spices, and Condiments
carob
cinnamon
clove
cumin
dill
garlic
ginger
mustard, with few ingredients
oregano
parsley
rosemary
tarragon
thyme
turmeric
vinegar

Sweeteners
Small Amounts
stevia, honey, maple syrup

Core Supplements for Lowering Inflammation and Supporting Your Gut

I have created a basic supplement program for you to stay on for the next six months or longer in order to continue the gut repair process, so that your gut bacteria can shift into a better balance that is resilient to outside life events that happen to us all. In addition, you will also continue to support your body to make less inflammation, which will keep your joints feeling their best. And we will also add a new joint repair supplement to help rebuild damaged joints.

The core long-term plan consists of both the omega oils, vitamin D, a multivitamin, L-glutamine, and probiotics. You should stay on omega-3 (EPA and DHA) and omega-6 (GLA) at the same high dose that you started at the beginning of the Arthritis Protocol, but in six months, when you finish step 3, you can cut the dose in half. You should stay on the curcumin, but you can drop the dose to 500 milligrams daily and have the option of continuing with the vitamin C, as you should be eating plenty of antioxidants in your new food plan. There is one new supplement that you should add for step 3, and that is undenatured type 2 collagen, because the studies are promising for its ability to repair joints in people with both rheumatoid arthritis and osteoarthritis.

- omega-3 fish oil: 3 grams daily of EPA and DHA
- omega-6: 500 milligrams daily of GLA from evening primrose or borage oil
- vitamin D_3: 2,000 IU daily
- multivitamin with antioxidants: two capsules daily
- curcumin: 500 milligrams daily
- vitamin C: 1,000 milligrams daily (optional)
- undenatured type 2 collagen: 10 milligrams daily

Building Gut Health and Resiliency

The gut environment is influenced by all kinds of damaging behavior, and for permanent, deep repair, it is critical to identify and reduce these behaviors. I will show you how. The goal is to "grow" good bacteria. Taking probiotics offers only a transient improvement, so other approaches are needed as well. For both your well-being and your gut, you need to understand the direct influence that stress, ingested toxins such as pesticides and GMO foods, alcohol, medication, and foods like processed sugar, smoked meats, a high intake of animal products, and so on have on the gut microenvironment. Following these guidelines is critical for shifting the terrain of your gut environment to one of health instead of disease. They must be incorporated into a long-term lifestyle change, not just a two-month treatment program. I already laid out the food plan and basic supplements; now let's look specifically at what your gut needs for deeper repair.

The first two months of a gut cleanse are an important jump-start, but they don't cause a permanent shift of the gut bacteria. This must be followed by sustained gut support that slowly shifts the terrain of the body. While following the Healthy Eating Plan and taking your basic supplements, you will also need to support the gut in a few simple ways. Here are your most important foundational supplements for the first year:

1. **Glutamine Powder**. I recommend staying on 4 to 5 grams (roughly one teaspoon) of glutamine powder per day. The loose powder is easy to use: just mix with water on an empty stomach or ten to fifteen minutes before eating. Glutamine will help heal the leaky gut and improve the strength of your intestinal lining. You can also add it to a protein shake or smoothie.

2. **Probiotics**. I already shared with you the best choices of probiotics in step 2, the Two-Month Intensive Gut Repair, and as you now move into deeper healing, you should increase the dose to at least 50 billion daily of a good mixed-strain formula. You can try going up to 100 billion and see if you develop digestive symptoms such as gas and gurgling. If you do, then cut back to the lower dose of 50 billion.

3. **Digestive Enzymes**. It is hard to know if you still need the enzymes, so you should stop them for a few weeks and notice if

any digestive symptoms come back, such as constipation, gas, bloating, and reflux. If so, stay on them and check again in two to three months to see if you still need them. Eventually you will be able to stop.

4. **Gut Cleanse**. At the end of step 3, the Finish-What-You-Started Six-Month Program, it will likely be necessary to repeat the gut cleanse for another thirty days. If your gut symptoms have returned or your arthritis continues to flare up, or your improvement seems to have plateaued even while following the rest of the program, another month of herbs is recommended. Most people, like June and Sherry, need to repeat the gut cleanse every six months until they were fully recovered. Do not view this as a failure; it is to be expected and is the way that you will *finish what you started*.

Summary of Your Step 3 Supplement Program

Basic Supplements
- omega-3 fish oil: 3 grams daily of EPA and DHA
- omega-6: 500 milligrams daily of GLA from evening primrose or borage oil
- vitamin D_3: 2,000 IU daily
- curcumin: 500 milligrams daily (new dose)
- multivitamin with antioxidants: two capsules daily
- vitamin C: 1,000 milligrams daily (optional)

Gut Repair Supplements
- digestive enzymes: one or two with each meal (optional)
- probiotics: 50 billion to 100 billion CFU daily (new dose)
- L-glutamine powder: one teaspoon daily (new dose)

Joint Support
- undenatured type 2 collagen: 10 milligrams daily

Suggested Schedule

Supplement	With Breakfast	With Lunch or Dinner
fish oil capsules	2	2
GLA capsules	I	I
omega liquid (alternative to fish oil and GLA capsules)	I tablespoon daily	
multivitamin with antioxidants	2	
vitamin D$_3$		I
curcumin	I	
vitamin C	I	
Soothe protein powder	I–2 scoops	
probiotics	I	I
digestive enzymes	I	I with lunch and I with dinner
L-glutamine powder	I teaspoon	
undenatured type 2 collagen	I	

Mind-Body Practice for Treating Trauma and Stress

Chances are, the stressors in your life have a greater effect on your health than you realize. Or maybe you *do* realize it but don't know what you can do about it and have just accepted it. I can't tell you how many people walk into my office every day and tell me that they had a flare-up in their symptoms, and they know exactly why it happened: stress. Whether taking care of a sick or dying person, or coping with a series of deadlines at work, having financial stress, or trying to manage difficult teenagers, these things make up the fabric of everyday life, and they affect us all unless we are very mindful and very, very careful. And sometimes there are traumatic events to deal with, such as physical or sexual abuse, or a fear of safety, as happened to me when I was robbed in Mexico City.

Stress has a profound physical effect on the body, and it specifically damages the gut bacteria and intestinal lining. Since repairing the gut is the focus for healing your arthritis, preventing this stress effect is a crucial part of your program. Also, stress wreaks havoc deep inside the inner terrain of your body, and since our other main goal is to build resiliency and shift your terrain to a healthy place, you must begin to create a bulletproof vest that will protect you from these stress effects. The way you create this is by starting and maintaining some kind of relaxation practice every day. We want the stress to bounce off you and not cause you harm.

This is the trifecta for getting and staying healthy: food, stress, and gut. These are the lifestyle pieces that need vigilance, commitment, and discipline, or you will not get fully, permanently better. Period. I promise, though, that it isn't as hard as you might think, and my job is to help you find a mind-body practice that you like and can do. Ready? Here goes.

Understanding the Mind-Body-Spirit Connection

Understanding my definition of the mind-body-spirit connection will help you understand how mind-body exercises work. Your mind is the part of you that is always thinking, planning, worrying. We are continuously bombarded with memories of the past and worries about the future, and these thoughts have the power to create a strong emotional reaction in the body, similar to what I described happens with post-traumatic stress disorder. The image you create in your mind with your thoughts triggers the same reaction in your body as if you are *actually* experiencing it in real time. Now, that is powerful!

The mind-body connection is understanding that your feelings, thoughts, and emotions get translated into your body. Stressful or traumatic memories, anger, and anxiety are examples of thoughts that exert a negative physical effect. What if you could take a break from these thoughts? When you practice mindfulness and mind-body exercises such as meditation, this helps bring your attention to *this moment*, so that you aren't thinking about the past or future. Actually, the ultimate goal is to take a break from thinking at all. This is the antidote that we all need.

Harnessing the power of this mind-body connection gives you a break from the incessant chatter in your mind and helps your body relax, not only while you're doing the exercises. Over time, and with daily (or at least most days) practice, you will find that the mindfulness you cultivate while practicing spills over into the rest of the day, and you will feel more relaxed, and less reactive to situations and people around you. And this translates into feeling less stressed.

An added bonus to practicing a mind-body exercise regularly is that it also will open you up to your mind-body-spirit connection. When I speak of spirit, I am referring to the intuition or inner voice that we all have deep inside us. I often refer to this inner voice as the North Star that each of us possesses: ever present and available to answer our deepest questions and guide us through life. The problem is that while we are busy rushing around and cluttering our minds by thinking all the time, we can't hear this intuitive voice above all the noise. Practicing mind-body exercises helps quiet your mind, so that you will start feeling this connection and can hear your own intuition giving you good advice. I can't tell you how many times during the quietest of moments meditating, an inspiration comes to me, and I just know it is the solution to something I had been thinking about. This is not the same as meditating and trying to come up with a solution. Instead, in the quiet of *not* thinking, you make space to really get to know yourself. I call this process "checking in."

Many people love to watch TV as a way to relax. This is fine, but it is a form of checking *out*, similar to getting lost on the computer or playing video games. It might take your mind off your worries, but as soon as you turn off the TV, your thoughts and concerns come flooding back, once again causing you stress. When you check in with mind-body exercises, you become aware of all the emotions, thoughts, and feelings that might be bottled up inside you, which you can think of as increasing your internal temperature. Most of the time we aren't even aware that we have this *heat* stuck inside us. By becoming aware of it, this heat actually bubbles up and is released, allowing you to *cool off*, so that your stress lifts and goes away. Connecting deep inside to your intuition is how you develop your mind-body-spirit connection, which has been a very powerful guide for me throughout my adult life and helped me through my most difficult times. In addition, it has helped me make many important business decisions building and growing Blum Center for Health.

Remember, a stressor is something *external* that has the potential to cause you to *experience* stress. You can't always change your stressors, but you can prevent yourself from feeling stressed by frequently checking in with yourself as you continue to follow a regular mind-body practice. I want you to think of these mind-body practices as a form of exercise. There are many different kinds, some of which you can do on your own, while others are better done with a group or teacher. Many can be followed and learned online or by using an app, and I will give you those resources. And, just like developing an exercise routine, these mind-body practices must be experienced to have the desired effect on your body. You can't sculpt your muscles just by *reading* about running or push-ups, and the same goes for mind-body practices. They are what we call *experiential,* so you must do them. After a few months of your new routine, it will simply become part of your life. But to get started will require discipline and commitment, and this is really the only way to change your terrain and *finish what you started.* Otherwise you run the risk of having a flare-up every time you experience something stressful. Remember Jorge, the young Haitian man with rheumatoid arthritis who finally started to really improve once he started meditating every day? As a result, he was able to reduce the amount of prescription medication he was taking. This is something that I see very frequently with my patients, not just those with autoimmune disease or arthritis.

One such patient had struggled for years to lose weight. Stacey, a forty-five-year-old teacher, went to the gym almost every day and followed a healthy anti-inflammatory diet, but she also had a lot of stress at work, lived alone, and always struggled to be truly happy in her life. She started ballroom dancing three nights each week, truly immersing herself in the music and dance, and found connection and joy in a new community of friends. Within four months, she had lost twenty pounds and was happier than I had ever seen her.

Bringing Mindfulness to Your Daily Life

There are many mind-body options. First, I will talk about those that you can do yourself and might already be doing. Then we'll review all the different options that you can do on your own but with the help of a teacher (whom you can find online, through an app, or from a workshop). If you are new to mindfulness, these exercises are best learned by experience, and this means following someone's voice or being guided in some way in real time. Instead of providing you with written exercises, I will tell you where to find a virtual teacher with a live voice and the guidance you need to get started. Finally, we will discuss finding a therapist or healer to help you relax your mind by working on your body.

You might not realize that simple things you are already doing, such as daily prayer, knitting, or walking the dog, can be a mind-body exercise if you follow a few simple guidelines. The idea is to bring mindfulness into the activity so that it becomes relaxing and opens you up to checking in with yourself. Here are some ideas and suggestions:

- When going for a stroll or walking the dog, leave your phone home or turned off and put away. Notice the leaves, gardens, wind, and small animals that live around your neighborhood.
- Pay attention to your sleep habits. Turn off electronics for at least thirty minutes before going to sleep and give yourself a bedtime. I recommend going to sleep no later than eleven o'clock and aiming for a minimum of seven hours' sleep each night. This is an important time for internal repair work to your stress system.

If you have trouble falling asleep, try an Epsom salts bath to relax your body and quiet your mind. A bath in the evening is a perfect opportunity to practice relaxation and meditation.

- Pay attention to what you are doing while you are commuting to and from work, and use the time on the train or in the car as an opportunity for a mindfulness practice. While driving, do not listen to the news and instead listen to music or an uplifting book on tape. If you are on the train, consider downloading an app. (See "Mind-Body-Spirit Exercises" on page 251 for suggestions.) These are all timed meditations, so you won't miss your stop on the train. Just put on your headphones, close your eyes, and follow the instructions. This is especially great for the ride home, when you want to transition from the busy day to a more relaxed state of mind.

- If you have a creative hobby such as knitting, painting, or writing, you can set an intention to make this time more mindful by turning off your phone, the computer, and other distractions so that you can focus 100 percent on your activity. The goal is to disengage from the constant stream of thoughts coming from your mind, and, by focusing on another relaxing activity, your mind and body will relax. But you must think of these hobbies as your mindfulness practice and not multitask while doing them.

- Many people tell me that exercise is their way to relax. I am very enthusiastic about the importance of daily exercise and activity, especially in people with every kind of arthritis, who benefit greatly from daily movement. However, most people multitask while exercising, talking to friends on the phone, watching TV, reading, or listening to loud, distracting music. This is not a mindful way to exercise. To use exercise as your mind-body-spirit practice, you need to create a focus: like your breath, or if you are outside, observing nature. Outdoor exercise is especially conducive to a meditative experience. I always feel that exercise is good for "clearing out my head" and is a great stress reliever. However, for connecting to your inner intuition and checking in with yourself, it isn't as effective unless you are distraction free while doing it.

- Prayer is one of the first types of meditation ever created by man. Many people say the rosary, for example, when they wake up or go to sleep, and don't realize this is meditating! If you are inclined toward using prayer as your meditation, just make it a formal commitment by deciding on a time and place in your home where you will practice every day.

Mind-Body-Spirit Exercises

The following is my list of different exercises you can learn and the resources to find guidance, whether through an app, a website, a video, or a teacher or workshop. I will share with you the advantages of each and my personal experience teaching and trying them all. My suggestion is that you try many different things until you find one that you like best.

Movement

Moving meditations are great for releasing trauma from the body and also if you are anxious or have a very jumpy mind and find it hard to sit still.

Yoga is probably the most common form of moving meditation and very easy to find both in your community and online. Ideally, joining a group and going to class offers the support that many people really enjoy. However, since most of us can't do this every day, the online option makes daily practice more affordable and convenient. There is everything from beginner to advanced classes, with varying degrees of instruction and lengths of time, and by trying a few sites and teachers, you are sure to find something that you like. If you believe that your arthritis pain will be a problem, I encourage you to try to do what you can, since the movement can help open up and bring lubrication to your joints. Some of the online offerings are free, and some have a subscription. Here are some options:

- YogaGlo, www.yogaglo.com
- Gaia, www.gaia.com
- Free on YouTube, examples:
    - Kino Yoga, www.youtube.com/user/KinoYoga
    - Yoga by Candace, www.youtube.com/user/YOGABYCANDACE
    - Yoga with Adriene, www.youtube.com/user/yogawithadriene
- Apps:
    - Pocket yoga
    - Sworkit

Tai chi is a Chinese martial art and form of meditative exercise characterized by methodically slow, circular stretching movements and positions of bodily balance. Its cousin, Qigong, is an ancient Chinese health care system that integrates physical postures, breathing techniques, and focused intention. I know many people who practice these and swear by their mind-body-spirit benefits. I recommend finding a teacher, a workshop, or a class, or you can travel to one of the retreat centers that I have listed below.

Dance classes such as Zumba or ballroom dancing can be a wonderful way to take a holiday from thinking and to focus on movement. However, to use these as your mindfulness practice, you would need to practice them at home, too, almost every day. I often tell my patients to put on music and dance around their bedroom while getting dressed in the morning. Or dedicate five to ten minutes to closing your eyes and letting loose before getting in the shower. This is a wonderful way to start your day and very easy to add to your daily routine.

Osho Dynamic Meditation is a moving meditation I learned from the Center for Mind-Body Medicine, and have taught and practiced it for almost twenty years. It is based on the teachings of a yogi named Osho and was apparently developed at meditation camps in the Indian mountains in the 1970s. His prototypical method is still named Dynamic Meditation and is available online. These are tremendously effective for working with trauma, and I used Dynamic Meditation to treat myself after I was robbed at gunpoint in Mexico and to release my overwhelming anxiety after my son's head injury. There is a tradition of these kinds of movement in ancient cultures such as the Sufis, who meditate while whirling and spinning in rhythmic movements. To find free Osho instructional videos, go to its website at www.osho.com/meditate. You can stream music conducive to practicing Dynamic Meditation at New Earth Records (www.new earthrecords.com/music/osho-dynamic-meditation).

Meditation and Guided Visualization

These mind-body practices are usually done sitting or lying down. There are many classical types of meditation that you might have heard of, such as Buddhist or yoga meditation, but the simplest to learn is easily found on apps that appeal to a broad audience. These free apps are favorites of my patients, and you can customize the length of your breathing, meditation, or visualization session. They are also portable and can be done on the plane, train, or during your lunch break at work:

- Headspace
- Calm
- Stop, Breathe, and Think

There are numerous Buddhist traditions, such as Vipassana, Zen, and Transcendental Meditation. Rather than think of these as classes, people practice together in community groups called *sanghas*, which are defined as Buddhist communities of monks, nuns, novices, and everyday people. They are very welcoming to anyone wanting to learn to meditate. In every city, you can find a *sangha* to join and start your meditation practice with lots of support. They also offer retreats and online teachings. My cousin is a Zen practitioner, and this was the first kind of meditation that I learned, more than twenty years ago. Since then, I tend to lean more toward Vipassana because it has less chanting and no rules about how to sit and eat. I also have done many trainings with wonderful teachers. The following websites for workshops and resources can get you started:

- Insight Meditation Society, www.dharma.org
- Zen Buddhism, www.zen-buddhism.net/practice/zen -meditation.html
- Transcendental Meditation, www.tm.org

In addition to Buddhist communities, there are also Indian yoga communities that practice meditation, often called self-realization meditation. You might remember that in the movie *Eat, Pray, Love,* Julia Roberts's character goes to an ashram in India. The community that she joined is real and is called the Siddha Yoga Path, led by Gurumayi Chidvilasananda, the Siddha Yoga guru. There are wonderful, free meditations that you can experience on its website, and a welcoming community to join if you are inclined. There is also a wonderful online community led by Gangaji, an American-born and Indian-taught spiritual teacher. These are good if you want to learn a more spiritually based meditation. I have had the extraordinary pleasure of attending retreats with both Gangaji and the Siddha Yoga community, and these experiences have woven their way into the fabric of my meditation practice:

- Siddha Yoga Path, www.siddhayoga.org
- Gangaji, gangaji.org

Then there are some great meditation teachers, styles, and trainings that grew out of the Buddhist tradition but were born and developed in America for the average person to learn. The most commonly known and offered program was developed by Jon Kabat-Zinn, Ph.D., at the University of Massachusetts Medical School. He developed a Mindfulness-Based Stress Reduction (MBSR) course that is open to the public and also trains teachers who then offer this eight-week course in the communities where they live and work. You have the option of taking the course online, attending a retreat for a concentrated one-week experience, or joining a group run by an MBSR teacher in your community.

- MBSR Online Course, www.soundstrue.com/store/mbsr-course.
- Mindfulness-Based Stress Reduction, Center for Mindfulness in Medicine, Health Care, and Society, University of Massachusetts, www.umassmed.edu/cfm/stress-reduction. Take the course where it all started.
- To find a teacher in your area where you can go to a class, visit www.umassmed.edu/cfm/stress-reduction/find-an-mbsr-program.
- Omega Institute offers several different versions of this course in a retreat setting, www.eomega.org.

Finally, another great organization that offers all types of meditation is the Center for Mind-Body Medicine. I have been working at CMBM since 1998. It is where I learned to both teach and practice all of these mindfulness exercises that I am sharing. As a faculty member, I have used the skills that it teaches to help people with everyday stress and to work with traumatized populations both here in the United States and in Haiti. If you are a health professional, you can go to its trainings to learn these techniques for yourself, but for everyone else, you can find someone trained and certified by CMBM in your community to work with and learn from. They also have many online resources, listed below. Also, Elizabeth Greig, our wonderful nurse practitioner at the Blum Center for Health, is certified by CMBM and has recorded an audio of eight different mind-body exercises similar to the ones used in that program, which you can find on BlumHealthMD.com/product/learn-relax-toolkit, called *Learn to Relax Tool Kit*.

- Center for Mind-Body Medicine, www.cmbm.org/ (general information).
- www.cmbm.org/self-care/ (free guided videos for meditation, imagery, and visualization).
- www.blumhealthmd.com/product/learn-relax-toolkit (audio guide with eight different meditation and guided imagery exercises).

Bodywork

If you are struggling to begin a meditation or other mind-body practice that starts with the mind relaxing the body, another option is to begin with the body as a way to relax the mind. This is what I refer to as bodywork. This is a very effective way to start, and often, over a few months' time, you can begin to think about beginning and including one of the other self-care practices that you would do on your own. Bodywork can include a broad range of therapeutic options, including massage, acupuncture, reiki, and craniosacral therapy. Sometimes there is overlap: for example, my acupuncturist is also trained in craniosacral therapy and works on my head and neck while the needles are applied and doing their magic. While this might not sound enjoyable, I assure you that by the end of the session, I am deeply relaxed and feeling balanced—almost melting on her table and needing to be peeled off when we are done! Finding a great hands-on therapist can be life changing and certainly something that I recommend as part of your Finish-What-You-Started Six-Month Program. You need to find all the ways to balance your stress system and shift your terrain. A good bodyworker can help you do this.

Unfortunately, most of these practitioners are not covered by insurance, although some plans do reimburse for acupuncture. If you have a health savings account as part of your insurance plan, you can pay for it with this money. It is well worth it. Usually the best way to find these practitioners is by referral, so ask your friends, your local spa, gym, or yoga center, for recommendations. Here are some guidelines:

- **Acupuncture**. Make sure they are licensed, and, ideally, trained in Traditional Chinese Medicine, and that they check your pulse and your tongue at your first session, because this will confirm that they are using Chinese Medicine to diagnose your condition and then prescribe your treatment. Unfortunately, there is no specific school or graduate program that determines the best people, so you will need to rely on your own experience to decide if the person is right for you.

- **Craniosacral Therapy**. The Upledger Institute International has been training people since 1985. You can search its database at www.upledger.com to learn more and find a practitioner in your community.

- **Massage Therapy**. There are many kinds of massage, and you should choose one that you find relaxing, not painful. The idea is to help your body relax, which will naturally quiet your mind.

- **Reiki Therapy**. This is a type of energy medicine that can help your body heal and relax. If possible, find a certified Reiki master, which means that the person has achieved the highest level of training.

Talk Therapy

I truly believe in getting all the support you can during difficult times. Many people benefit from finding someone to talk to about their worries, family relationships, and stressors. You can find a therapist who has a master's degree in social work, a master's in psychology, a Ph.D.-trained psychotherapist, and others. There are many different approaches that you can choose, including traditional talk therapy, cognitive behavioral therapy (CBT), and somatic experience therapy (SE). I have become a big fan of SE and want to tell you a little more about it.

Somatic experience, an approach to healing trauma and traumatic stress, was founded by a therapist named Peter Levine, Ph.D. He wrote several great books, including *In an Unspoken Voice: How the*

Body Releases Trauma and Restores Goodness, and his colleague, Bessel van der Kolk, M.D., wrote another great book called *The Body Keeps the Score: Brain, Mind, and Body in the Healing of Trauma.* Somatic experience therapists teach you mind-body techniques such as breathing and grounding exercises (feeling your feet on the floor helps to bring you back into the present moment) that you can use when you are consumed by anxiety, stress, and worry. It is especially effective for treating PTSD. I believe mind-body exercises like this can help you release the trauma and stress from your body, thus supporting the health of your inner terrain, which is such a key puzzle piece to reduce systemwide inflammation and have a healthy gut. It is great to have a teacher who can show you how to do this and help you connect the dots between how you feel and how your body is reacting. There are several SE therapists that I am connected to in my community, and I send them referrals very often because the work they do with my patients is really helpful. One of my patients had a young daughter with cancer, and even though her daughter survived, the experience left my patient with panic attacks every time she walked into a hospital. After working with an SE therapist for a few months, the panic attacks were gone, because she had developed strategies and tools to manage the situation. Find a practitioner in your community at the Somatic Experiencing Trauma Institute, http://sepractitioner.membergrove.com.

Residential Retreats and Centers

Over the past fifteen years, I have attended at least a dozen different retreats and workshops around the country to hone my mind-body-spirit connection. These workshops were (and still are) open to the public, and I went to many different programs, ranging from silent meditation retreats to a weekend practicing Sufi meditation and dancing. The place that I went most often was the Omega Institute for Holistic Studies, in Rhinebeck, New York. It was like going to camp, with a communal vegetarian dining hall and simple accommodations, all reasonably priced. I recommend going to a place like this if you want to jump-start your mind-body practice, have a deeper experience with a group of like-minded people, or enhance your home practice. There are several places in the New York area where I live, but there are also options around the country. Think of it as going on a self-care vacation! On a typical vacation, you often return home feeling toxic from all the alcohol and food you ate while away; on a self-care vacation, you come home balanced, refreshed, and with new additions to your healthy tool kit. Here are some suggestions:

- Omega Institute for Holistic Studies, www.eomega.org
- Kripalu Center for Yoga and Health, https://kripalu.org
- Spirit Rock for Insight Meditation, www.spiritrock.org

Working with Your Doctor to Taper Your Medication

As we come to the end of the Arthritis Protocol and *Healing Arthritis,* I want to leave you with some advice about tapering your medication. You need to do this with your doctor, never by yourself. It doesn't matter if your physician understands or even approves of the Arthritis Protocol; all that matters is that he or she sees that you are better. Your labs will have improved, and your symptoms, too, which will open the door to the discussion about changing your medication. I encourage you to share what you've been doing and your commitment to continue with the program, so that your doctor feels confident that you won't relapse if you lower your medication. Remember, your doctor's focus is on making sure that you don't relapse and suffer joint damage, so this reassurance that you are committed to the program is key to gaining his or her support.

Keep in mind, you might not be ready yet to taper your medication by the end of the Arthritis Protocol. It is hard to predict this, because it depends on how severe your arthritis and condition were when you started. I hope that the patients' stories that I have shared with you have illustrated the many ways that this can unfold. The most important thing I want to leave you with is hope and a road map of where to go next. Some of you might need to work through the

Arthritis Protocol only one time, but my experience is that you will need to repeat step 2's Intensive Gut Repair every six months or so, as your gut microbiome and intestinal lining are slowly and completely healed. Your joints will slowly and surely heal, too. Because many people do need guidance to figure out what comes next, you can find online support from my team at www.blumhealthmd.com.

CHAPTER 11

Recipes

Chef Amy Bach created the majority of these delicious and simple recipes that are designed to follow both the Leaky Gut Diet for Arthritis and the Healthy Eating Plan. Those labeled "Organic Pharmer" were contributed by Lee and Darleen Gross, executive chefs and culinary directors of Organic Pharmer grab-and-go health food eateries in Rye Brook and Scarsdale, New York, which I cofounded because my patients were clamoring for prepared food that would make it easier for them to stick with an anti-inflammatory diet.

Breakfast Recipes

Applesauce Cranberry-Almond Muffins
Recipe makes 12 muffins

3 cups almond flour

2 teaspoons cinnamon

½ teaspoon nutmeg, grated

1 teaspoon lemon zest

¼ teaspoon salt

¼ cup coconut sugar

¼ cup honey

1 teaspoon vanilla extract

1 tablespoon sunflower oil

2 flax eggs (2 tablespoons ground golden flax mixed with ¼ cup plus 6 tablespoons water; mix and set aside)

¾ cup unsweetened applesauce

½ cup fruit-juice-sweetened dried cranberries, chopped

½ cup dried apples, chopped

Directions
1. Preheat oven to 325 degrees.
2. Lightly grease 12-cup muffin pan.
3. In a large mixing bowl, whisk almond flour, spices, and salt.
4. In a medium mixing bowl, whisk coconut sugar, honey, vanilla, sunflower oil, flax eggs, and applesauce until well blended.
5. Add wet mixture to the dry mixture and stir until combined.
6. Fold in cranberries and dried apples.
7. Divide the batter equally into prepared muffin cups.
8. Bake for 25 minutes.
9. Rotate and bake an additional 5 minutes.
10. Let cool in pan for 10 minutes before removing.

Organic Pharmer's Power Porridge
Recipe makes 1 quart, or 3 to 4 servings

A few notes:
- The quinoa can be replaced with other gluten-free grains such as millet, amaranth, teff, or buckwheat.
- To speed up cooking and improve digestibility, soak grains in the water overnight.
- Instead of water, you can use almond, rice, or coconut milk, or you can pour the milk over the cooked porridge at the table. Your toppings allow you to tailor it to your taste as well as add nutrition to your bowl.

1 cup gluten-free rolled oats
¼ cup quinoa
1 tablespoon brown flaxseed, toasted

1 pinch sea salt
3 cups filtered water

Directions
1. Combine the oats, quinoa, flaxseed, salt, and water in a pot and bring to a boil.
2. Reduce heat to low, cover, and simmer gently for 20 to 25 minutes.
3. Remove from heat and add your choice of toppings, such as: roasted walnuts, sunflower seeds, raisins, goji berries, dried tart cherries, fresh berries, sliced bananas, chopped apples, pears, peaches, or plums when in season, cacao nibs, toasted coconut flakes, a drizzle of honey or maple syrup, and a dusting of cinnamon or grating of fresh nutmeg.

Organic Pharmer's Coconut Golden Milk
Recipe makes 4 cups

1 can full-fat coconut milk

2 cups filtered water

2 cinnamon sticks

4 whole cloves

1 teaspoon green cardamom
   pods, crushed

½ teaspoon black
   peppercorns

1 teaspoon turmeric, ground

2 teaspoons orange zest

2 tablespoons fresh ginger,
   chopped roughly

¼ teaspoon vanilla extract

2 tablespoons raw honey (or to
   taste)

Directions

1. Combine all ingredients except vanilla and honey in a saucepan and bring to a boil.
2. Turn heat to medium-low, cover, and simmer gently for 10 to 15 minutes.
3. Remove from heat, strain, and stir in vanilla and honey.
4. Serve warm or chilled, or use in hot tea or coffee.

Juices

Organic Pharmer's Anti-Inflammatory Elixir
Recipe makes one 6- to 8-ounce glass of juice

3 large carrots, peeled
1 green apple
1 small cucumber, peeled
2-inch piece fresh gingerroot

4-inch piece fresh turmeric root
1 pinch black pepper, freshly
   ground

Directions
1. Wash the fruits and vegetables well.
2. Pass them through a centrifugal or cold-pressed juicer to extract juice.
3. Whisk in pepper and serve immediately.

Main Dishes

Adzuki Bean Burger with Warm Spices
Recipe makes 4 to 6 burgers

1 cup dried sprouted adzuki beans, soaked overnight and cooked for 40 minutes with ½ teaspoon baking soda (Baking soda helps reduce the gas factor associated with beans.)

½ cup scallions, green tops only, sliced finely

2 flax eggs (2 tablespoons ground golden flax mixed with ¼ cup plus 6 tablespoons water; mix and set aside)

½ cup carrots, scrubbed and finely shredded

½ cup zucchini, shredded, with excess water squeezed out

2 tablespoons sunflower seeds, toasted and finely ground

½ cup quinoa, cooked

1 teaspoon fresh ginger, minced

½ teaspoon coriander, ground

½ teaspoon cumin, ground

½ teaspoon turmeric, ground

Salt and pepper to taste

1 tablespoon oil of choice

Directions

1. Preheat oven to 375 degrees.
2. Mash ½ of the cooked adzuki beans in a large mixing bowl.
3. Add remaining whole beans and the rest of the ingredients.
4. Form into 4 to 6 equal-sized patties.
5. Lightly grease sheet pan with ½ of the oil and place the formed burgers on the pan. Rub the remaining oil on the tops of the burgers. (This will help with the browning process and give a slight crust to the burger.)

6. Bake for 30 minutes or until golden brown and a crust has formed on the burgers.
7. Remove from oven and let rest 5 minutes before removing from pan.
8. Eat right away or let cool, wrap in parchment paper, and freeze.

Rich Bean, Vegetable, and Quinoa Burgers
Recipe makes 6 burgers

1 15-ounce can of cannellini beans or "meaty" bean of choice, drained

2 tablespoons lemon juice

1 cup tricolor quinoa, cooked

½ cup red onion, finely diced

½ cup spinach, cooked, chopped, excess water squeezed out (frozen is fine)

½ cup zucchini, shredded, excess water squeezed out

1 teaspoon granulated garlic

1 teaspoon dried thyme

½ teaspoon sea salt

¼ teaspoon black pepper, freshly ground

⅓ cup gluten-free oat flour

2 flax eggs (2 tablespoons ground golden flax mixed with ¼ cup plus 6 tablespoons water; mix and set aside)

Sunflower oil for frying or extra-virgin olive oil for baking the burgers

Directions

1. If baking burgers in oven, preheat to 375 degrees.
2. In a small bowl, using a fork or your hands, mash beans, leaving a few beans whole with lemon juice.
3. In a large mixing bowl, add quinoa, mashed beans, onion, spinach, zucchini, garlic, thyme, salt, and pepper and mix well.
4. Add in oat flour and flax eggs and mix well again.
5. Refrigerate for about 1 hour for mixture to set up. It will be easier to form patties if mixture is cold.
6. Form into 4 to 6 equal-sized burgers. If mixture sticks to your hands, dampen your hands with cold water.
7. Cooking option 1: Brush burgers with extra-virgin olive oil on both sides, place on oiled sheet pan, and bake for 30 minutes, flipping burgers halfway through cooking.
8. Cooking option 2: Heat about 3 tablespoons sunflower oil in a

skillet until hot but not smoking, add burgers, and fry until golden brown, turning once.

9. Serve with favorite toppings.
10. These can be frozen.

Baked Cod with Chermoula Sauce
Recipe makes 4 servings

Chermoula is a traditional Moroccan sauce/marinade usually used on fish. It also can be used on vegetable, bean, and grain dishes. I have removed 1 teaspoon of paprika and ⅛ teaspoon of cayenne from the recipe since these are nightshades; feel free to add them if you can tolerate them.

Olive oil for greasing the sheet pan

4 pieces of firm, white fish fillets (6 to 7 ounces each) such as cod, halibut, mahi-mahi, or other fish of choice

Salt and black pepper to taste

Lemon wedges for serving

Chermoula Sauce
Recipe makes 1 cup

2 cups picked cilantro leaves (about two bunches)

1½ cups flat leaf parsley

½ teaspoon sea salt

3 to 4 medium cloves of garlic, grated on a microplane

2 teaspoons cumin seeds, lightly toasted and ground in a spice grinder for best flavor *or* prepared ground cumin

½ teaspoon coriander seeds, toasted and ground on a spice grinder *or* prepared ground coriander

¼ cup fresh lemon juice

½ cup extra-virgin olive oil

Directions

1. Preheat oven to 350 degrees.
2. In a food processor bowl, add all of the ingredients except for the olive oil.
3. Mix until a paste forms, add olive oil, and mix well. Remove from processor and set aside.
4. Lightly grease a sheet pan with extra-virgin olive oil.
5. Place fish fillets in a large bowl. Salt and pepper the fillets and add a rounded ¼ cup of Chermoula Sauce, coating the fish on all sides using your hands.
6. Place the fish on the prepared sheet pan and bake for 20 to 25 minutes, depending on the thickness of the fish.
7. Remove from pan and serve with lemon wedges and the remaining Chermoula Sauce on the side. (Chermoula Sauce can be refrigerated for one week or frozen for two months.)

Ginger Miso Glazed Salmon
Recipe makes 4 servings

This dish goes well with Forbidden Black Rice Pilaf in the "Grains" on page 277.

4 salmon fillets (6 to 7 ounces each), wild caught preferred. Check fillets for small "pin bones" and remove.

1 tablespoon chickpea miso or mung bean miso (available in Whole Foods refrigerated section)

1½ tablespoons gingerroot (more or less to taste), minced

1 tablespoon mirin cooking wine (available in the Asian section of most supermarkets)

2 tablespoons coconut amino acids (available in Whole Foods, by the soy sauce)

½ teaspoon toasted sesame oil

1 teaspoon Sucanat or organic raw sugar of choice

1 tablespoon sesame seeds for garnish (optional)

3 scallions, thinly sliced on the diagonal, for garnish (white and light-green parts only)

Directions
1. Preheat oven to 375 degrees.
2. Rinse fish in cold water and pat dry.
3. Line a sheet pan with parchment paper and place salmon fillets on parchment.
4. In a medium mixing bowl, combine miso, ginger, mirin, coconut aminos, sesame oil, and sugar and use a small whisk to combine well.
5. Pour or brush marinade over fish and bake for 20 to 25 minutes, depending on your desired doneness.
6. Remove pan from oven and use a spatula to place fish on a serving platter or plate.
7. Pour pan sauce over fish and garnish with sesame seeds and scallions.

Tuscan Kale and Shallot-Stuffed Chicken Breasts
Recipe makes 4 servings

2 packed cups (about 1 bunch) of cooked chopped Tuscan kale (also known as lacinato kale or dinosaur kale), center ribs removed

2 tablespoons of extra-virgin olive oil, plus 2 teaspoons, divided

½ cup shallots, peeled, sliced

2 small cloves garlic, smashed and minced

3 tablespoons Kalamata olives, chopped (optional)

2 teaspoons lemon zest

2 tablespoons pine nuts, toasted (optional)

½ teaspoon sea salt

½ teaspoon black pepper, freshly ground

4 chicken breasts with skin

1 teaspoon fresh rosemary, chopped

Directions

1. Preheat oven to 375 degrees.
2. Cook kale: in a large saucepan, bring 4 cups of water to a boil, add chopped kale, and simmer for about 7 minutes until tender. Pour out water over a strainer and then rinse kale under cold water to retain bright-green color. Squeeze out excess water and chop well.
3. In a small skillet, heat 2 tablespoons of olive oil over medium-high heat, cook shallots for 5 to 7 minutes until soft and slightly golden.
4. Add garlic and cook 5 minutes longer.
5. Add chopped Kalamata olives (if using), lemon zest, chopped cooked kale, pine nuts (if using), and salt and pepper to taste.
6. Stir well and remove from heat.

(*continued on next page*)

7. When filling is cool enough to handle, divide into 4 equal portions. Set aside.

8. Take chicken breasts and gently loosen skin under one side with your index finger, creating a "pocket" for the filling.

9. Gently place one portion of filling under loosened skin. Pull skin over breast and tuck under. Repeat with remaining breasts.

10. Rub 2 teaspoons of olive oil on chicken breasts and season tops and bottoms with salt and pepper.

11. Sprinkle tops of chicken breasts with rosemary and place chicken breasts on a small sheet pan skin side up.

12. Bake in preheated oven for 30 to 40 minutes depending on size.

13. Remove from oven and let sit for 10 minutes. Be sure to reserve the pan juices to pour over chicken when serving.

Loaded Turkey Meatloaf
Recipe makes 6 to 8 servings

3 tablespoons extra-virgin olive oil

1½ cups yellow onion, finely chopped

2 teaspoons thyme, dried

2½ pounds ground turkey meat, preferably a 50/50 mixture of thigh and breast meat

2 flax eggs (2 tablespoons ground golden flax meal plus 6 tablespoons water combined, stirred, and set aside)

¼ cup flat leaf parsley, chopped

1 can cannellini beans, rinsed and drained

1 packed cup spinach (frozen is fine), cooked, chopped; squeeze out excess water

½ teaspoon sea salt

½ teaspoon black pepper, freshly ground

2 tablespoons of Dijon mustard, plus 2 teaspoons, divided

Directions
1. Preheat oven to 350 degrees.
2. Lightly grease an 8 x 4-inch loaf pan and set aside.
3. Heat 2 tablespoons olive oil in a small skillet and sauté onions and thyme for about 7 minutes over medium-high heat until translucent.
4. Remove onions from pan and let cool.
5. In a large mixing bowl, combine turkey meat, flax eggs, cooked onions, parsley, cannellini beans, spinach, the remaining tablespoon of olive oil, salt, pepper, and 2 tablespoons of the Dijon mustard and mix thoroughly.
6. Place turkey mixture into greased loaf pan and spread remaining 2 teaspoons of Dijon mustard over top.

(*continued on next page*)

7. Put a sheet pan under the loaf pan before baking in case of juice overflow.
8. Place in oven and bake for 1 hour.
9. Let sit in pan for 15 minutes before serving.
10. This can be enjoyed cold as a sandwich meat.

Grains

Forbidden Black Rice Pilaf
Recipe makes 4 servings

2 cups water
1 cup forbidden black rice
1 teaspoon sea salt
1 tablespoon sunflower oil
6 scallions, trimmed and
  thinly sliced
2 tablespoons fresh
  gingerroot, peeled and
  finely minced

3 cups sugar snap or snow peas,
  trimmed and cut into 1-inch
  pieces
1 tablespoon rice wine vinegar
3 tablespoons cilantro, chopped

Rice

Directions
1. In a medium saucepan with a lid, bring water to a boil.
2. Add rice and 1 teaspoon of salt and bring to a boil.
3. Turn heat down to a simmer and cook covered for about 25 to 30 minutes.
4. Turn off heat, keep covered, and let steam for 10 minutes.
5. Fluff with a fork.
6. Keep covered until vegetables are ready.

Sugar snap or Snow Peas

Directions
1. In a large skillet, heat the sunflower oil over medium-high heat for about 2 minutes.

(continued on next page)

2. Add scallions and ginger and cook for 5 minutes, stirring occasionally.
3. Add the sugar snap or snow peas and cook an additional 3 minutes.
4. Add cooked black rice, rice wine vinegar, and cilantro and stir to combine.
5. Add salt to taste.
6. Serve immediately or let cool and have a cold rice salad.

Vegetable Confetti Quinoa
Recipe makes 4 to 6 servings

3 cups water

1½ cups tricolor quinoa

1 teaspoon sea salt

3 tablespoons extra-virgin
olive oil ½ cup

½ cup red onion, diced
small

1 cup carrots, peeled and
diced small

1 small green squash, seeded
and diced small

1 small yellow squash, seeded
and diced small

½ teaspoon salt, plus salt and
pepper to taste

½ cup fresh parsley leaves,
loosely packed

¼ cup fresh mint leaves, loosely
packed

Directions

1. Add the water, quinoa, and ½ teaspoon of salt to a medium saucepan and bring to a boil.
2. Cover and reduce to a low simmer for about 15 minutes or until all water is absorbed.
3. Turn off heat and set the saucepan aside, covered.
4. In a large skillet, heat the olive oil over a medium-high flame until pan is hot.
5. Add onions and cook for 5 minutes, stirring occasionally.
6. Add carrots, green squash, yellow squash, salt, and pepper.
7. Stir and cook for 5 minutes more.
8. Add fluffed quinoa, parsley, and mint and stir well to combine.
9. Serve immediately or let cool and enjoy as a cold dish.

Wild Rice Pilaf with Dried Cherries and Pecans
Recipe makes 4 to 6 servings

2 tablespoons sunflower oil or ghee (clarified butter)

1 cup wild rice

1 cup short-grain brown rice

3 large shallots, peeled and minced

1 bay leaf

2 sprigs fresh thyme or ¼ teaspoon dried thyme

½ teaspoon sea salt

4 cups chicken or vegetable stock

½ cup dried fruit-juice-sweetened cherries, chopped

⅓ cup pecans, toasted and chopped (Toast in a 350 degree oven on a sheet pan for about 5 minutes. Caution: Nuts have a high oil content and can burn quickly, so be careful!)

¼ cup flat leaf parsley, chopped

Black pepper, freshly ground

Directions
1. In a medium stockpot, heat sunflower oil or ghee for 5 minutes.
2. Add wild rice, brown rice, and shallots and stir to coat with oil or ghee.
3. Cook until shallots are soft, about 3 minutes.
4. Add bay leaf, thyme, salt, and stock and bring to a boil.
5. Cover and reduce to a simmer for about 40 to 50 minutes or until all liquid is absorbed.
6. Remove from stove and stir in cherries, pecans, parsley, salt and pepper to taste.
7. Serve hot or cold.

Vegetable Dishes

Zucchini "Pasta" with Green Harissa Sauce
Recipe makes 4 to 6 servings

Traditional harissa is a fiery hot sauce from Tunisia. This toned-down recipe has all the flavor without the heat of the peppers.

Green Harissa Sauce

1 packed cup flat leaf parsley leaves
½ cup cilantro leaves
¼ cup mint leaves
2 medium cloves garlic

Juice from half a lemon
1 teaspoon cumin, ground
⅓ cup extra-virgin olive oil
½ teaspoon sea salt
Black pepper, freshly ground

Directions
1. Place all ingredients in a blender except the olive oil and blend until smooth.
2. With the blender running, slowly add the oil until incorporated.
3. Add the salt, and pepper to taste.
4. Remove from blender and set aside.

Zucchini "Pasta"

2 tablespoons extra-virgin olive oil
3 scallions, trimmed and thinly sliced
1 cup fresh or defrosted frozen baby peas

3 cups shaved or "spiralized" zucchini (If you don't have a spiralizer, use a vegetable peeler and peel long, thin strips of zucchini.)

(*continued on next page*)

2 cups baby spinach, stems
  trimmed

Sea salt and black pepper,
  freshly ground

Directions

1. Heat olive oil in a large skillet over medium heat until hot, about 3 minutes.
2. Add scallions and peas and sauté for about 3 minutes. (If using frozen peas, cook for 1 minute.)
3. Stir in zucchini and baby spinach and cook for 5 minutes longer.
4. Add salt and pepper to taste.
5. Add Green Harissa Sauce and stir well to mix sauce throughout the vegetables.

Cauliflower Couscous with Currants and Toasted Almonds
Recipe makes 4 to 6 servings

1 large head of cauliflower, cut into small florets (discard the tough center core)

1 to 2 tablespoons extra-virgin olive oil

Sea salt and freshly ground black pepper to taste

⅓ cup currants

¼ cup sliced almonds, toasted (Toast in a 350 degree oven on a sheet pan for about 5 minutes. Caution: Nuts have a high oil content and can burn quickly, so be careful!)

2 tablespoons flat leaf parsley, finely chopped

Directions

1. Preheat oven to 375 degrees.
2. Place half the cauliflower in bowl of a food processor and pulse into a uniform course meal; remove and repeat with the remaining cauliflower.
3. Remove cauliflower from food processor and put on paper towels to remove excess water.
4. In a large mixing bowl, combine cauliflower, olive oil, salt, and pepper and mix well.
5. Place cauliflower on a sheet pan and bake in oven for 12 minutes, stirring once.
6. Remove cauliflower from oven and add currants, almonds, and parsley and stir to combine.
7. Remove from pan and serve.

Maple Roasted Brussels Sprouts and Butternut Squash
Recipe makes 4 to 6 servings

1 large butternut squash
(about 3 pounds), peeled
and cut into 1½-inch dice
1 pound Brussels sprouts,
trimmed and cut in half
½ teaspoon sea salt

½ teaspoon black pepper, freshly
ground
2 tablespoons extra-virgin olive
oil
2 tablespoons maple syrup

Directions
1. Preheat oven to 400 degrees.
2. In a large mixing bowl, combine the butternut squash, Brussels sprouts, salt, pepper, olive oil, and maple syrup and toss well to coat.
3. Place mixture on a sheet pan or two, so as not to crowd vegetables during roasting. Bake for 25 minutes.
4. Remove from oven and serve.

Haricot Verts/Green Beans with Shallots and Lemon
Recipe makes 4 to 6 servings

1½ pounds haricot verts or green beans, ends trimmed

2 medium shallots, peeled and thinly sliced

1 rounded teaspoon lemon zest

1 to 2 tablespoons extra-virgin olive oil

Sea salt and black pepper, freshly ground

Directions

1. Preheat oven to 400 degrees.
2. Place the beans, shallots, and lemon zest on a sheet pan and stir to combine.
3. Drizzle with olive oil and stir again.
4. Add salt and pepper to taste.
5. Bake for 20 to 25 minutes.
6. Remove from pan and serve.

Snacks

Goji Berry Nut and Seed Energy Bars
Recipe makes 12 bars

1 cup walnuts
½ cup almonds
½ cup sprouted pumpkin
 seeds
8 dates, pitted, chopped,
 soaked in hot water
1 tablespoon sunflower oil
2 tablespoons coconut flour
1 teaspoon vanilla extract
½ cup maple syrup

3 tablespoons pumpkin protein
 powder
½ teaspoon sea salt
1 cup goji berries
¼ cup mini chocolate chips,
 soy and dairy free (Enjoy Life
 brand is a good choice.)
½ cup unsweetened coconut,
 shredded, dried

Directions
1. Preheat oven to 350 degrees.
2. Lightly grease an 8 x 8-inch cake pan and line with parchment paper so that it hangs over the edge of the pan. (The overhang will make it easier to remove the bars from the pan when they're done.)
3. Place walnuts, almonds, and pumpkin seeds on a sheet pan and toast in the oven for 7 minutes.
4. Remove nuts and seeds from the oven and let them cool. Keep the oven on.
5. Drain dates and discard water.
6. In a food processor, grind nuts and seeds into a rough meal, not powder.
7. Add dates, sunflower oil, coconut flour, vanilla, maple syrup, pumpkin protein powder, and salt and pulse until just combined.
8. Remove the mixture from the food processor, put it into a bowl, and stir in goji berries, chocolate chips, and shredded coconut.

9. With wet fingers, evenly press the mixture into the cake pan.
10. Bake for 20 minutes.
11. Remove from oven and let cool for 10 minutes.
12. Remove bars from pan and let them cool completely.
13. Cut cooled bars into 12 or more equal portions and peel off parchment paper.
14. Store in an airtight container in the refrigerator.

Red Beet Hummus Snack
Recipe makes 4 to 6 servings

1 medium red beet, peeled and cut into large dice shapes, about 1½ cups total

¼ cup extra-virgin olive oil

Sea salt and black pepper, freshly ground

½ teaspoon lemon zest

2 or more tablespoons fresh lemon juice

2 small cloves garlic, minced

2 tablespoons tahini

1 15-ounce can garbanzo beans, drained and rinsed

¼ cup walnuts, toasted (optional)

Directions

1. Preheat oven to 375 degrees.
2. Toss diced beets with 1 teaspoon olive oil, salt, and pepper and place on sheet pan.
3. Roast until soft, about 25 minutes.
4. Remove from the oven and let cool.
5. In a food processor, add beets, lemon zest, lemon juice, garlic, and tahini and pulse until smooth, scraping down sides.
6. Add drained garbanzo beans, walnuts (if using), salt, and pepper and pulse to combine.
7. Add the remaining olive oil and some water and blend until creamy and smooth. (Add more water if necessary to thin out.)
8. Scrape out of food processor with a rubber spatula and chill before serving.
9. Enjoy with vegetables and gluten-free crackers of your choice.

Sweet and Spicy Crunchy Chickpeas
Recipe makes 6 servings

2 15-ounce cans garbanzo beans/chickpeas, drained and rinsed

2 tablespoons extra-virgin olive oil

1 tablespoon fresh lemon juice

1 teaspoon coconut sugar

1 teaspoon maple syrup

1½ teaspoons cumin, ground

½ teaspoon coriander, ground

¼ teaspoon cinnamon, ground

1 teaspoon garam masala (an Indian spice)

½ teaspoon black pepper, freshly ground

½ teaspoon sea salt

Directions

1. Preheat oven to 400 degrees.
2. In a large mixing bowl, combine chickpeas, olive oil, and lemon juice; stir well to coat chickpeas with the liquid.
3. In a small bowl, mix together all the spices with a small whisk or fork.
4. Add spices to the chickpeas and toss well to combine.
5. Put the chickpea mixture on a sheet pan in a single layer, being careful not to crowd the chickpeas. You want room around them so they can dry out and roast.
6. Place the sheet pan in the oven and bake for 35 to 45 minutes until the chickpeas are brown in spots, crisp, and shrunken. Stir at least once.
7. Remove from the oven and loosen the chickpeas from the pan with a spatula if necessary.
8. Let cool.
9. Store in an airtight container when completely cooled.

Herbed White Bean Dip
Recipe makes 4 servings

1 15-ounce can cannellini beans, drained and rinsed

2 medium cloves garlic, minced

¼ cup fresh lemon juice

½ teaspoon sea salt or pink Himalayan salt to taste

¼ teaspoon black pepper, freshly ground

⅓ cup extra-virgin olive oil

2 to 3 tablespoons water, for thinning the dip (use more or less if necessary)

1 tablespoon flat leaf parsley, chopped

2 tablespoons fresh dill, chopped

½ teaspoon fresh rosemary, chopped

1 tablespoon fresh chives, minced

Directions

1. Place drained cannellini beans, garlic, lemon juice, salt, pepper, and olive oil in the bowl of a food processor and pulse until smooth, adding water if needed. Adjust seasoning if needed.
2. Add chopped herbs and pulse *only* two times to mix, or you will get a green dip instead of a nice, herb-flecked dip.
3. Remove from bowl with a rubber spatula and serve.

Organic Pharmer's Carrot-Beet Cleanser
Recipe makes 3 to 4 servings

1 large carrot, peeled and
  coarsely grated

2 medium red beets, peeled
  and coarsely grated

Juice of 1 large orange

Juice of 1 lemon

½ teaspoon fresh ginger
  juice (grate ginger and
  squeeze juice from pulp)

1 tablespoon extra-virgin olive oil

½ teaspoon parsley, minced

¼ teaspoon mint, minced

Pinch of sea salt

Pinch of cayenne pepper

Directions
1. Combine all ingredients in a mixing bowl and toss.
2. Let sit for a few minutes to allow flavors to develop before eating.

Organic Pharmer's Spicy Black Bean Dip
Recipe makes about 1 quart

4 tablespoons extra-virgin
olive oil

2 cups Spanish or white
onion, chopped

3 cloves garlic, peeled
and chopped (about 1
tablespoon)

2 jalapeño peppers, chopped
(remove seeds for a less
spicy dip)

1 can black beans, rinsed
and drained (reserve
2 tablespoons beans for
garnish)*

1½ teaspoons sea salt (or to
taste)

½ teaspoon cumin, ground

¼ teaspoon coriander, ground

¾ teaspoon cayenne pepper
(or to taste)

3 tablespoons fresh lime juice

Water, as needed to thin

1½ tablespoons red onion,
minced

1 cup small cherry or grape
tomatoes, quartered

¼ cup cilantro plus 2
tablespoons, chopped

Directions

1. Heat the olive oil over medium heat in a small saucepan.
2. Add the onions, garlic, and jalapeño peppers and cook, stirring occasionally, until very soft, about ten minutes.
3. Transfer the onion mixture to a blender or food processor, add the black beans, salt, cumin, coriander, cayenne, 2 tablespoons lime juice and blend until smooth. Add water if needed to thin to desired consistency.
4. Taste and adjust seasoning.
5. Transfer to a serving bowl.

---

*Eden brand beans are recommended because they are certified organic, additive free, and cooked with kombu, a sea vegetable that adds valuable nutrients and makes them more digestible.

6. In a separate mixing bowl, combine red onion, the remaining lime juice, and salt to taste and let mixture sit for 10 minutes.
7. Fold in the chopped tomatoes, reserved black beans, and ¼ cup cilantro, spoon attractively onto the dip, and sprinkle the remaining 2 tablespoons of cilantro on top as garnish.
8. Serve with a crudité of fresh organic vegetables, including jicama, red bell peppers, and carrot sticks, or with your favorite chip.

Soups

Beef Bone Broth
Recipe makes about 2 to 3 quarts

A few important points:
- Use a selection of grass-fed beef bones, oxtails, ribs, and cut-up knuckles (have your butcher do this); they're especially good with a little meat on them.
- Blanch your beef bones by placing them in a large stock pot and covering with cold water. Bring to a boil and reduce to an aggressive simmer for 20 minutes. Remove bones and discard water. Bones are now ready for roasting!

4 to 5 pounds assorted grass-fed beef bones, blanched

4 medium carrots, scrubbed and roughly chopped

½ pound celery, coarsely chopped

2 medium yellow onions, peeled and coarsely chopped (Save onion skins for the stock; they add a rich color!)

6 to 8 large cloves of garlic, smashed

1 small bunch of Italian parsley, washed to remove grit and dirt

4 bay leaves

½ bunch fresh thyme

½ teaspoon black peppercorns

3 tablespoons apple cider vinegar

¼ ounce dried shiitake mushrooms

Salt to taste

Directions
1. Preheat oven to 450 degrees.
2. Place blanched bones on a sheet pan.
3. Put sheet pan in the oven and roast for 45 minutes.
4. Remove from the oven, add carrots, celery, and onions, and roast for 10 minutes.

5. Remove from the oven, add smashed garlic, and roast 5 more minutes.
6. Remove browned bones and vegetables and transfer to a large stockpot, scraping up all brown bits and liquids that have accumulated while roasting.
7. Add parsley, bay leaves, thyme, peppercorns, apple cider vinegar, dried shiitake mushrooms, and salt to taste.
8. Add enough cold water to just cover all the bones and bring to a boil over medium heat.
9. Reduce heat to a low simmer for at least 3 to 5 hours, occasionally skimming off foam and some fat from surface.
10. Remove pot from stove and strain stock through a fine mesh sieve over a large bowl or another stockpot, pressing down on solids.
11. Discard solids.
12. Let broth cool. Place the pot or bowl in an ice bath if you want to bring down the temperature quickly.
13. Cover and chill or freeze up to three months.

Chicken Bone Broth
Recipe makes about 4 quarts

These bones don't require blanching like the beef bones, but roasting is a must for great rich flavor!

5 pounds chicken neck bones, wings, feet (they have a high gelatin content), or any other chicken bones (You can save and freeze bones from roasts in your freezer for this stock.)

20 cups cold water, plus 1 cup

3 large carrots, scrubbed and roughly chopped

3 celery stalks with leaves, roughly chopped

2 large yellow onions with skin on, cut into quarters

4 cloves garlic, smashed

3 tablespoons apple cider vinegar

2 bay leaves

3 sprigs thyme

6 sprigs flat leaf parsley

1 teaspoon peppercorns

1 teaspoon pink Himalayan salt

Directions
1. Preheat oven to 375 degrees.
2. Place all the chicken bones on a sheet pan; possibly two pans so as not to crowd the bones.
3. Place in oven and roast for 40 minutes or until nicely browned.
4. Remove from oven and pour about 1 cup of water on pan to loosen browned bits; then scrape roasted chicken bones and browned bits into a large stockpot.
5. Add vegetables, apple cider vinegar, herbs, peppercorns, salt, and the remaining water.
6. Bring to a boil.

7. Turn down to a simmer and cook for 5 to 6 hours, occasionally skimming off foam and fat from top of broth.
8. Strain broth through a fine sieve over a large bowl or another stockpot, pressing on solids to release remaining juices.
9. Place in storage containers and freeze up to three months or refrigerate for one week.

Spiced Cauliflower Soup
Recipe makes 6 to 8 bowls

3 tablespoons coconut oil

1 medium onion, trimmed and thinly sliced

1 large fennel bulb, trimmed and thinly sliced

2-inch piece of fresh turmeric root, peeled and thinly sliced

2 stalks celery, trimmed and thinly sliced

2 teaspoons cumin, ground

1 teaspoon coriander, ground

½ teaspoon dried thyme

Sea salt and black pepper, freshly ground

1 large head cauliflower, cut into florets

8 cups (2 quarts) vegetable or chicken stock

Directions

1. In a large stockpot, heat coconut oil over medium-high heat.
2. Add the onions, fennel, turmeric root, celery, cumin, and coriander.
3. Cook for 10 minutes until fragrant.
4. Add dried thyme, salt and pepper to taste, cauliflower, and stock to pot.
5. Bring to a boil.
6. Reduce to a simmer for about 30 minutes or until the cauliflower is soft.
7. When soup is cool enough to handle, place small batches in a blender and puree until smooth.
8. Taste for salt and pepper, reheat, and serve.

Lentil and Root Vegetable Soup
Recipe makes 6 to 8 bowls

3 tablespoons olive oil

1 medium onion, thinly sliced

2 medium cloves garlic, chopped

3 celery stalks, trimmed and diced

3 medium carrots, scrubbed and diced

3 medium parsnips, peeled and diced

½ a small, red kuri squash or Delicata squash, peeled and diced

Salt and black pepper, freshly ground, to taste

3 sprigs fresh thyme

1 large bay leaf

1 quart vegetable or chicken stock

1 quart filtered water

1 cup French lentils that have been soaked for 3 hours and drained (Soaking aids in digestion and speeds cooking time.)

3 tablespoons flat leaf parsley, chopped

3 cups kale, spinach, or Swiss chard, chopped

Directions
1. Heat olive oil in a large stockpot over medium-high heat.
2. Reduce heat and add onions, garlic, celery, carrots, parsnips, and squash.
3. Cook for 7 minutes, stirring occasionally.
4. Add salt, pepper, thyme, and bay leaf.
5. Add stock and water to soup pot with vegetables.
6. Add drained lentils and bring to a boil.
7. Reduce heat and simmer soup for 25 minutes or until lentils are tender.
8. Remove thyme stems and bay leaf, add parsley and kale, spinach, or Swiss chard.
9. Simmer for 5 more minutes.

Detox Broth with Kombu and Shiitake Mushrooms
Recipe makes 6 to 8 bowls

2 tablespoons olive oil or coconut oil

1 medium onion, peeled and sliced

3 celery stalks with leaves chopped

2 medium carrots, peeled and sliced

3 medium cloves garlic, smashed

1 fennel bulb, trimmed and sliced

1 bay leaf

1 tablespoon whole coriander seeds

1 12-inch piece of Burdock root, also known as "GOBO," peeled and thinly sliced (found in Asian markets)

1 2-inch piece gingerroot, peeled and thinly sliced

1 2-inch piece turmeric root, peeled and thinly sliced

1 6-inch piece dried kombu

1 cup dried shiitake mushrooms

1 teaspoon black peppercorns

½ bunch flat leaf parsley

3 quarts filtered water

Sea salt

Directions
1. Add oil to a large 8-quart stockpot and cook over medium-high heat.
2. Add onion, celery, carrots, garlic, fennel, bay leaf, and coriander seeds.
3. Cook for about 7 to 10 minutes or until fragrant.
4. Add remaining vegetables, shiitake mushrooms, herbs, and 3 quarts of water.
5. Bring to a boil and then reduce to a simmer and cook covered for 1 hour or longer.
6. Strain soup liquid through a fine mesh strainer.
7. Discard other vegetables, saving shiitake mushrooms for slicing into the reserved broth.
8. Remove tough stems from cooked shiitake mushrooms and slice the caps thinly.
9. Add sliced mushrooms and salt to taste to strained broth and enjoy.

Creamy Celery Root Soup
Recipe makes 4 to 6 bowls

4 cups celery root, peeled and cut into large dice

2 cups carrots, washed and chopped

2 parsnips, peeled and chopped

1 tablespoon olive oil

Sea salt and white pepper

1 bouquet garni (2 bay leaves, 2 sprigs fresh thyme, 4 sprigs fresh parsley, and 2 sprigs fresh rosemary wrapped in a piece of cheesecloth and tied with kitchen twine)

1½ quarts chicken or vegetable stock

1 or 2 tablespoons nutritional yeast

Directions
1. Preheat oven to 375 degrees.
2. Place celery root, carrots, parsnips, olive oil, salt and pepper to taste in a large bowl. Toss well to coat with oil.
3. Place oiled vegetables on a sheet pan and place in the oven.
4. Roast for 25 minutes or until lightly browned in spots.
5. In a large stockpot, combine roasted vegetables, bouquet garni, stock of choice, and nutritional yeast.
6. Bring to a boil over high heat.
7. Reduce to a simmer until vegetables are soft.
8. Remove bouquet garni.
9. Carefully puree soup in a blender a little at a time until creamy and smooth. (Always use caution when blending hot soup!)
10. Salt and pepper to taste.
11. Serve hot or cold.

Salads

Bountiful Beet Chopped Salad with Lemon Tahini Dressing
Recipe makes 4 to 6 servings

1 bunch beets with fresh green tops attached (5 to 6 beets in a bunch)

1 tablespoon extra-virgin olive oil

Sea salt and black pepper, freshly ground

6 scallions, white and light-green parts only

1 pound baby kale mix or your favorite young greens

1 fennel bulb, trimmed and thinly sliced

Lemon Tahini Dressing (see recipe on page 303)

½ cup sunflower seeds, toasted

Directions
1. Preheat oven to 375 degrees.
2. Trim the tops off the beets, wash well, and discard tough stems and damaged leaves.
3. Cut remaining leaves into bite-sized pieces and set aside.
4. Peel and cut beets into large dice.
5. Toss with olive oil, salt and pepper to taste.
6. Place cubed beets on sheet pan.
7. Bake for 20 minutes or until just tender. (You don't want them soft!)
8. Remove cooked beets from the oven and place on a cold sheet pan to cool.
9. In a large salad bowl, combine cooled beets, beet greens, scallions, baby greens, and fennel. Toss with Lemon Tahini Dressing. Garnish with toasted sunflower seeds.

Lemon Tahini Dressing
Recipe makes 1 cup

¼ cup tahini (sesame seed paste)

¼ cup fresh lemon juice

2 tablespoons apple cider vinegar

2 tablespoons honey

1 small clove garlic, minced

¼ cup water

3 tablespoons extra-virgin olive oil

Sea salt and black pepper, freshly ground

Directions

1. Place tahini, lemon juice, vinegar, honey, garlic, and water in a blender and blend until creamy.
2. Add olive oil and more water if necessary to thin.
3. Add salt and pepper to taste.

Detox Confetti Salad with Turmeric Dressing
Recipe makes 4 to 6 servings

1 small head cauliflower, finely chopped in a food processor

1 small head broccoli, finely chopped in a food processor

2 carrots, peeled and shredded

1 cup flat leaf parsley leaves, chopped

½ cup sunflower seeds, toasted

¼ cup currants

2 cups curly kale, chopped

1 cup red cabbage, shredded

Turmeric Dressing (see recipe on page 305)

Directions
1. Place all ingredients in a large mixing bowl.
2. Top with Turmeric Dressing and serve immediately.

Turmeric Dressing
Recipe makes ½ cup

3 tablespoons fresh turmeric root, peeled and chopped

2 tablespoons tahini sauce

¼ cup extra-virgin olive oil

1 tablespoon coconut aminos

1 lemon, juiced (about 3 tablespoons)

1 teaspoon lemon zest

2 small cloves garlic, chopped (optional)

1 teaspoon nutritional yeast

1 teaspoon gingerroot, minced

2 teaspoons honey

Sea salt and black pepper, freshly ground

Directions
1. Place all ingredients in a blender and pulse until smooth.
2. Add a small amount of water to thin if necessary.
3. Add salt and pepper to taste.
4. Use immediately or refrigerate for one week.

Rainbow Asian Slaw
Recipe makes 4 to 6 servings

1 English hothouse cucumber, cut into thick 3-inch long matchstick pieces

6 scallions, trimmed and cut on the bias

2 medium-sized purple and yellow carrots also labeled as "rainbow carrots," peeled and grated on the large holes of a hand grater

½ head Napa cabbage, shredded (medium-sized head) with the tough center removed and discarded. This should yield about 5 to 6 cups.

2 to 4 tablespoons fresh mint, chopped; more or less to taste

½ bunch cilantro, chopped with tough stems removed and discarded

2 tablespoons coconut aminos

3 tablespoons toasted sesame oil

2 tablespoons sunflower oil

3 tablespoons rice wine vinegar

2 tablespoons maple syrup

2 teaspoons fresh ginger, peeled and grated

Sea salt and black pepper, freshly ground

2 tablespoons black and white sesame seeds for garnish

Directions

1. Place all prepared vegetables in a large serving bowl and toss well, using your hands.
2. In a small mixing bowl, whisk together coconut aminos, sesame oil, sunflower oil, rice wine vinegar, maple syrup, and ginger.
3. Add salt and pepper to taste.
4. Pour over slaw and toss well to combine.
5. Garnish with sesame seeds.

Very Veggie French Lentil Salad
Recipe makes 4 to 6 servings

2 cups carrots, peeled and cut into small dice

2 cups celery, trimmed and cut into small dice

2 cups French green beans (haricot verts), blanched and cooled, and then cut into ¼-inch pieces

1 cup flat leaf/Italian parsley leaves

3 tablespoons chives, chopped

2 cups French lentils, cooked

Dijon Dressing (see recipe on page 308)

Directions

1. Place all prepared vegetables, parsley, chives, and cooked lentils in a large serving bowl.
2. Stir to combine.
3. Set aside and prepare dressing.

Dijon Dressing
Recipe makes about 1 cup

2 tablespoons Dijon mustard
¼ teaspoon dried thyme
¼ cup white balsamic or
    champagne vinegar

1 teaspoon honey
½ cup extra-virgin olive oil
Sea salt and black pepper,
    freshly ground

Directions

1. In a small bowl, whisk together all the dressing ingredients until smooth.
2. Pour into lentil salad and mix well.
3. Adjust salt and pepper if necessary.

Desserts

Tropical Lime Chia Pudding
Recipe makes 6 servings

24-ounce can coconut milk
(lite is fine)
¼ cup honey
¼ cup maple syrup
Pinch of pink Himalayan salt
½ teaspoon vanilla extract
½ cup fresh pineapple,
finely chopped

1 teaspoon fresh lime zest
(microplaning works best)
2 to 3 tablespoons dried,
unsweetened coconut
¾ cup chia seeds

Directions

1. In a deep bowl, mix together coconut milk, honey, maple syrup, salt, vanilla, pineapple, lime zest, and coconut. Stir well.
2. Whisk in chia seeds and continue to whisk for about 5 to 10 minutes until pudding has thickened slightly and there are no clumps of chia.
3. Cover and refrigerate for at least two hours, until thick and chilled.

Seasonal Fruit Crisp
Recipe makes 6 servings

1 tablespoon tapioca starch
½ teaspoon vanilla extract
¾ cup coconut sugar, plus
  2 tablespoons
2 tablespoons fresh lemon
  juice
7 to 8 cups of seasonal fruits
  of your choice (In summer,
  try sliced peaches, plums,
  nectarines, blueberries,
  and blackberries; in the
  fall or winter, try sliced,
  peeled apples or pears.)

1 cup gluten-free oats
⅓ cup gluten-free oat flour
1½ teaspoons cinnamon
Pinch of pink Himalayan salt
⅓ cup sunflower oil

Directions
1. Preheat oven to 375 degrees.
2. Lightly grease a 9 x 9-inch cake pan.
3. In a medium mixing bowl, add tapioca starch, vanilla, 2 table-spoons coconut sugar, and lemon juice and mix well.
4. Add your fruit of choice and stir to combine.
5. Pour the fruit mixture into a cake pan and cover with plastic wrap.
6. In another bowl, add the oats, oat flour, cinnamon, salt, and the remaining ¾ cup coconut sugar, and stir well to combine.
7. Add the sunflower oil and stir until evenly moist and crumbly.
8. Refrigerate for 30 minutes.
9. Remove the plastic wrap from the fruit mixture and sprinkle the crumble mixture over it evenly.
10. Place in the oven and bake for 25 minutes.
11. Serve warm or cold.

Fruit Parfait with Coconut Whipped Cream
Recipe makes 4 servings

Note: Coconut milk must be refrigerated for 24 hours for it to whip properly.

1 chilled can full-fat coconut milk (lite coconut milk will not work)

2 tablespoons maple syrup

Pinch of pink Himalayan salt

¼ teaspoon vanilla extract

4 to 5 cups of fresh berries, peaches, or favorite fruit of choice

Directions
1. Open the can of coconut milk and drain the liquid. (You can save it to use in smoothies, soups, and curry sauce.)
2. Scrape out chilled coconut fat solids into a blender and add maple syrup, salt, and vanilla.
3. Blend well until whipped, occasionally scraping down sides.
4. Spoon your fruit of choice into a tall wineglass and top with whipped coconut cream.
5. Serve immediately and enjoy!

CONVERSION CHARTS

Oven temperature guide

	Electricity °C	Electricity °F	Electricity (fan) °C	Gas Mark
Very cool	110	225	90	$^1/_4$
	120	250	100	$^1/_2$
Cool	140	275	120	1
	150	300	130	2
Moderate	160	325	140	3
	170	350	160	4
Moderately hot	190	375	170	5
	200	400	180	6
Hot	220	425	200	7
	230	450	210	8
Very hot	240	475	220	9

Liquid measurements

Metric	Imperial	Australian	US
25ml	1fl oz		
60ml	2fl oz	¼ cup	¼ cup
75ml	3fl oz		
100ml	3½fl oz		
120ml	4fl oz	½ cup	½ cup
150ml	5fl oz		
180ml	6fl oz	¾ cup	¾ cup
200ml	7fl oz		
250ml	9fl oz	1 cup	1 cup
300ml	10½fl oz	1¼ cups	1¼ cups
350ml	12½fl oz	1½ cups	1½ cups
400ml	14fl oz	1¾ cups	1¾ cups
450ml	16fl oz	2 cups	2 cups
600ml	1 pint	2½ cups	2½ cups
750ml	1¼ pints	3 cups	3 cups
900ml	1½ pints	3½ cups	3½ cups
1 litre	1¾ pints	1 quart or 4 cups	1 quart or 4 cups
1.2 litres	2 pints		
1.4 litres	2½ pints		
1.5 litres	2¾ pints		
1.7 litres	3 pints		
2 litres	3½ pints		

Weight measurements

Metric	Imperial
10g	½ oz
20g	¾ oz
25g	1 oz
40g	1½ oz
50g	2 oz
60g	2½ oz
75g	3 oz
110g	4 oz
125g	4½ oz
150g	5 oz
175g	6 oz
200g	7 oz
225g	8 oz
250g	9 oz
275g	10 oz
350g	12 oz
450g	1lb
700g	1lb 8 oz
900g	2lb

Conclusion

I hope this book has taught you that while there are many different types of arthritis, the ongoing pain you are experiencing can be
treated without medication by finding and resolving the root cause
of your inflammation. Therefore, to truly heal arthritis, we focus on
strategies to repair the gut and adopt a long-term, gut-supporting lifestyle that includes eating a microbiome-friendly, anti-inflammatory
diet; improving sleep; reducing stress; getting regular exercise; and
increasing self-awareness of your body, mind, and spirit.

Clearly, *Healing Arthritis* is not a quick fix but instead a course cor-
rection in how you have been living your life. You will probably need
to give up some of your favorite habits, and I admit there will be some
sadness and grief over this. That's okay. Feel it, let it go, and then
move on. After all, it's worth it to reduce the severe joint pain that's
probably been holding you back from doing many things you want to
do and to have more energy to live your life more fully. This choice is
yours. But now you know that *you do have a choice* and that you can
heal arthritis, the number one cause of disability worldwide.

In addition to the do-it-yourself program in *Healing Arthritis*, I
have created a robust and supportive website at BlumHealthMD.com
that offers guidance and help as you go through the steps in this book.
We have a health coach standing by to answer your questions, and
this is all free, confidential, and available to anyone who needs it. I
have also created a 90-Day Arthritis Action Plan, which translates the

Arthritis Protocol into a week-by-week online program designed to give you all the tools you need for success. This program includes a personal health coach, an arthritis support group on Facebook, and all the supplements you need to follow the Arthritis Protocol.

Remember, every healing journey must begin with the first steps, and then to really *heal* arthritis, you must finish what you started. This book and program offer you the jump-start, then show you what comes next, including how to make permanent changes that will help you continue your journey toward a permanent cure. I know that you can do it, and I believe that you now have the tools for your success.

Acknowledgments

The saying "no man is an island" holds especially true when you're writing a book! From the earliest stages of birthing the idea, through the shaping of the manuscript, and then finally marketing and launching the book, I have been surrounded by truly wonderful people. They not only helped me with the book itself but also supported me in the rest of my life so that I had the space and time to research and write.

First and foremost, I am forever grateful for my husband, Bruce, my greatest champion, the wind beneath my wings. As the years roll by, I continue to feel blessed for his steadfast support in everything I do. I am one lucky gal. I also want to thank my three sons, Jeremy, Corey, and Avery, for understanding my preoccupation with writing and the time commitment required to birth a book. My boys always inspire me to reach for my dreams, just as I am encouraging them. I am one lucky mom.

As for writing the book itself, my greatest thanks and appreciation go to Michele Bender, who manages to turn my perhaps overly scientific writing and explanations into user-friendly dialogue that is easy to read and understand. Our writing relationship was born when we worked on *The Immune System Recovery Plan*. I think this book was easier for both of us because Michele's voice was already inside my head. I still hear her telling me to explain what I mean over and over! Thank you, Michele, for helping not only with the writing but also for always being available to turn material around quickly and for advice when I was stuck.

This book would not have been possible without my wonderful patients—especially those who allowed their stories to be shared in these pages. Thanks also to the many, many patients whom I have gotten to know and had the privilege to help. You helped me create the plan that we are now able to share with so many others who need it.

I also want to thank my agent, Janis Donnaud, for her constant support, ready answers to my questions, and for championing my cause. Shannon Welch, my editor at Scribner, was very easy to work with and I truly appreciate how enthusiastic she was about this book from the beginning. And a special acknowledgment and thanks to Roz Lippel and Susan Moldow at Scribner for their commitment to me and making sure I had everything I needed to bring *Healing Arthritis* to life. Scribner has taken good care of me!

I couldn't have written this book while also running Blum Center and seeing patients without the full support of my entire team. My eternal and tremendous gratitude goes to Cindy Conroy. You are more than my sister; you are my partner in all our business ventures, the CFO of Blum Center, and I couldn't possibly be where I am today without you. My other right-hand person is Sabrina DeGregorio, our center manager. I appreciate you more than you know. Thank you to my fellow clinicians at Blum Center, Elizabeth Greig, Darcy McConnell, Mary Gocke, Pamela Yee, and more recently Sezelle Gereau, Bronwyn Fitz, and Melissa Rapoport. You all keep me grounded and our work together has laid the foundation for the Arthritis Protocol that we now share with so many deserving people. And finally, Gary Goldman and Elspeth Beier, you have been with me since the beginning and I am so grateful for your big hearts, generous spirit, and warm counsel when I needed it.

I am forever grateful for the opportunity that I had to work with the Center for Mind-Body Medicine in their domestic training programs and in the Global Trauma Relief Program in Haiti. My experiences have shaped who I am and taught me everything I know about stress and trauma. Specifically, thank you to James Gordon, M.D., for being my greatest mentor, and my colleagues Kathy Farah, Jerrol Kimmel, Kelsey Menehan, Lynda Richtsmeier-Cyr, and Amy Shinal for always being there to support me, with a special shout-out to Toni Bankston, who opened my eyes to the effects of early childhood trauma on illness later in life.

Over the past few years, we have continued to work hard to get the word out about what we are doing at Blum Center through newsletters, digital platforms, social media, and marketing. Thank you to Sara Santora for keeping track of everything and working so diligently to help me launch all my new projects and to our newer team members from Digital Natives, Weston Gardner and Jonathan Jacobs. This past year I have been hard at work launching a new and expanded digital platform at BlumHealthMD.com, and Maria DiSalvo has been my rock as director of Blum Digital. Thank you, Maria! Your job hasn't been easy but you handle it all very gracefully. I couldn't have gotten the new website up with the 90-Day Arthritis Action Plan without you by my side. I am grateful for your dedication and hard work.

I have a big extended family and felt them all behind me as I wrote this book, trying to balance work and home. There are too many of you to thank individually, but I want to specifically acknowledge Carol Blum, my partner and cofounder of Organic Pharmer, for helping me in all the ways that matter.

And finally, I want to thank my parents for nurturing the belief inside me that I could do anything I put my mind to. My mother, Barbara Spanton, is my biggest fan, and my dad, who passed since I wrote my first book, still smiles down and encourages me forward.

Notes

Chapter 1: Rheumatoid Arthritis

1. S. Nikolaus et al., "Fatigue and Factors Related to Fatigue in Rheumatoid Arthritis: A Systematic Review," *Arthritis Care & Research* 65, no. 7 (July 2013): 1128–46.

2. I. E. Cock et al., "The Potential of Selected Australian Medicinal Plants with Anti-Proteus Activity for the Treatment and Prevention of Rheumatoid Arthritis," *Pharmacognosy* 11, no. 42 (supplement 1) (April–June 2015): S190–S208.

3. R. A. Ataee et al., "Simultaneous Detection of Mycoplasma Pneumoniae, Mycoplasma Hominis, and Mycoplasma Arthritidis in Synovial Fluid of Patients with Rheumatoid Arthritis by Multiplex PCR," *Archives of Iranian Medicine* 18, no. 6 (June 2015): 345–50.

4. Kerstin Klein and Steffen Gay, "Epigenetics in Rheumatoid Arthritis," *Current Opinion in Rheumatology* 27, no. 1 (January 2015): 76–82.

5. C. Ciccacci et al., "Polymorphisms in STAT-4, IL-10, PSORS1C1, PTPN2, and MIR146A Genes Are Associated Differently with Prognostic Factors in Italian Patients Affected by Rheumatoid Arthritis," *Clinical & Experimental Immunology* 186, no. 2 (November 2016): 157–63.

6. Sue Ellen Verbrugge et al., "Proteasome Inhibitors as Experimental Therapeutics of Autoimmune Diseases," *Arthritis Research & Therapy* 17, no. 1 (2015): 17.

7. Somaiya Mateen et al., "Increased Reactive Oxygen Species Formation and Oxidative Stress in Rheumatoid Arthritis," *PLoS ONE* 11, no. 4 (April 4, 2016): doi:10.1371/journal.pone.0152925.

8. Celia Maria Quiñonez-Flores et al., "Oxidative Stress Relevance in the Pathogenesis of Rheumatoid Arthritis: A Systematic Review," *BioMed Research International* (May 31, 2016): doi:10.1155/2016/6097417.

9. S. J. S. Flora, Megha Mittal, and Ashish Mehta, "Heavy Metal Induced Oxidative Stress & Its Possible Reversal by Chelation Therapy," *Indian Journal of Medical Research* 128, no. 4 (October 2008): 501–23.

10. Jose U. Scher et al., "Periodontal Disease and the Oral Microbiota in New-

Onset Rheumatoid Arthritis," *Arthritis & Rheumatology* 64, no. 10 (October 2012): 3083–94; Clifton O. Bingham III and Malini Moni, "Periodontal Disease and Rheumatoid Arthritis: The Evidence Accumulates for Complex Pathobiologic Interactions," *Current Opinion in Rheumatology* 25, no. 3 (2013): 345–53.

11. M. K. Söderlin et al., "Smoking at Onset of Rheumatoid Arthritis (RA) and Its Effect on Disease Activity and Functional Status: Experiences from BARFOT, a Long-Term Observational Study on Early RA," *Scandinavian Journal of Rheumatology* 40, no. 4 (2011): 249–55.

12. Jennifer H. Humphreys et al., "The Incidence of RA in the UK: Comparisons Using the 2010 ACR/EULAR Classification Criteria and the 1987 ACR Classification Criteria. Results from the Norfolk Arthritis Register," *Annals of the Rheumatic Diseases* 72, no. 8 (August 2013): 1315–20.

13. Dario Scublinsky and Claudio D. Gonzalez, "Quantifying Disease in Challenging Conditions: Incidence and Prevalence of Rheumatoid Arthritis," *Journal of Rheumatology* 43, no. 7 (July 2016); 1263–64.

14. Klein and Gay, "Epigenetics in Rheumatoid Arthritis."

15. Victoria H. Wilkinson, Emma L. Rowbotham, and Andrew J. Grainger, "Imaging in Foot and Ankle Arthritis," *Seminars in Musculoskeletal Radiology* 20, no. 2 (April 2016): 167–74.

16. Arnd Kleyer et al., "High Prevalence of Tenosynovial Inflammation Before Onset of RA and Its Link to Progression to RA—A Combined MRI/CT Study," *Seminars in Arthritis & Rheumatism* 46, no. 2 (October 2016): 143–50.

17. E. Suresh, "Diagnosis of Early RA: What the Non-specialist Needs to Know," *Journal of the Royal Society of Medicine* 97, no. 9 (September 2004): 421–24.

18. Ibid.

19. Yvonne P. M. Goekoop-Ruiterman et al., "Comparison of Treatment Strategies in Early Rheumatoid Arthritis: A Randomized Trial," *Annals of Internal Medicine* 146, no. 6 (March 20, 2007): 406–15.

20. Verbrugge et al., "Proteasome Inhibitors as Experimental Therapeutics."

21. Kiran Farheen and Sandeep K. Agarwal, "Assessment of Disease Activity and Treatment Outcomes in Rheumatoid Arthritis," *Journal of Managed Care Pharmacy* 17, no. 9 (supplement B) (November/December 2011): S9–S13.

22. Judith Haschka et al., "Relapse Rates in Patients with Rheumatoid Arthritis in Stable Remission Tapering or Stopping Antirheumatic Therapy: Interim Results from the Prospective Randomised Controlled RETRO Study," *Annals of the Rheumatic Diseases* 75, no. 1 (January 2016): 45–51.

23. Maria Pilar Lisbona et al., "ACR/EULAR Definitions of Remission Are Associated with Lower Residual Inflammatory Activity Compared with DAS28 Remission on Hand MRI in Rheumatoid Arthritis," *Journal of Rheumatology* 43, no. 9 (September 2016): 1631–36.

24. Laure Gossec, Maxime Dougados, and William Dixon, "Patient-Reported Outcomes as End Points in Clinical Trials in Rheumatoid Arthritis," *RMD Open: Rheumatic & Musculoskeletal Diseases* 1, no. 1 (April 22, 2015), e000019.

Chapter 2: Spondyloarthritis

1. DoQuyen Huynh and Arthur Kavanaugh. "Psoriatic Arthritis: Current Therapy and Future Approaches," *Rheumatology* 54, no. 1 (January 2015): 20–28; Gleison Vieira Duarte, César Faillace, and Jozélio Freire de Carvalho, "Psoriatic Arthritis," *Best Practice & Research: Clinical Rheumatology* 26, no. 1 (February 2012): 147–56.
2. Wilkinson, Rowbotham, and Grainger, "Imaging in Foot and Ankle Arthritis"; Jose Inciarte-Mundo et al., "Calprotectin and TNF Trough Serum Levels Identify Power Doppler Ultrasound Synovitis in Rheumatoid Arthritis and Psoriatic Arthritis Patients in Remission or with Low Disease Activity," *Arthritis Research & Therapy* 18, no. 1 (July 8, 2016): 160.
3. L. E. Durham, L. S. Taams, and B. W. Kirkham, "Psoriatic Arthritis," *British Journal of Hospital Medicine* 77, no. 7 (July 2016): C102–C108.
4. Durham, Taams, and Kirkham, "Psoriatic Arthritis."
5. Huynh and Kavanaugh, "Psoriatic Arthritis"; Duarte, Faillace, and de Carvalho, "Psoriatic Arthritis."

Chapter 3: Osteoarthritis

1. Giuseppe Musumeci et al., "Osteoarthritis in the XXIst Century: Risk Factors and Behaviours That Influence Disease Onset and Progression," *International Journal of Molecular Sciences* 16, no. 3 (March 2015): 6093–112.
2. Chelsea M. Clinton et al., "Whole-Foods, Plant-Based Diet Alleviates the Symptoms of Osteoarthritis," *Arthritis* 2015 (2015): doi:10.1155/2015/708152.
3. Ibid.
4. Yuqing Zhang and Joanne M. Jordan, "Epidemiology of Osteoarthritis," *Clinics in Geriatric Medicine* 26, no. 3 (August 2010): 355–69.
5. Ibid.
6. Musumeci, "Osteoarthritis in the XXIst Century."
7. Zhang and Jordan, "Epidemiology of Osteoarthritis."
8. Musumeci, "Osteoarthritis in the XXIst Century."
9. Richard F. Loeser, John A. Collins, and Brian O. Diekman, "Ageing and the Pathogenesis of Osteoarthritis," *Nature Reviews: Rheumatology* 12, no. 7 (July 2016): 412–20.
10. Musumeci, "Osteoarthritis in the XXIst Century."
11. K. H. Collins et al., "Relationship Between Inflammation, the Gut Microbiota, and Metabolic Osteoarthritis Development: Studies in a Rat Model," *Osteoarthritis and Cartilage* 23, no. 11 (November 2015): 1989–98.
12. Tuhina Neogi and Yuqing Zhang, "Epidemiology of Osteoarthritis," *Rheumatic Disease Clinics of North America* 39, no. 1 (February 2013): 1–19.
13. Stefanie N. Hofstede et al., "Variation in Use of Non-surgical Treatments Among Osteoarthritis Patients in Orthopaedic Practice in the Netherlands," *BMJ Open* 5, no. 9 (September 9, 2015): e009117.
14. M. M. Saw et al., "Significant Improvements in Pain After a Six-Week Physiotherapist-Led Exercise and Education Intervention, in Patients with

Osteoarthritis Awaiting Arthroplasty, in South Africa: A Randomised Controlled Trial," *BMC Musculoskeletal Disorders* 17, no. 1 (2016): 236.

15. Fulya Bakilan et al., "Effects of Native Type II Collagen Treatment on Knee Osteoarthritis: A Randomized Controlled Trial," *Eurasian Journal of Medicine* 48, no. 2 (June 2016): 95–101.

Chapter 4: Other Arthritis Conditions

1. Josef S. Smolen, "Undifferentiated Early Inflammatory Arthritis in Adults," UpToDate, last modified November 29, 2016, www.uptodate.com/contents /undifferentiated-early-inflammatory-arthritis-in-adults?source=preview&search =percent2Fcontentspercent2Fsearch&anchor=H366390521#H366390521.
2. Carol M. Greco, Thomas E. Rudy, and Susan Manzi, "Adaptation to Chronic Pain in Systemic Lupus Erythematosus: Applicability of the Multidimensional Pain Inventory," *Pain Medicine* 4, no. 1 (April 2003): 39–50.
3. Adrian Budhram et al., "Anti-cyclic Citrullinated Peptide Antibody as a Marker of Erosive Arthritis in Patients with Systemic Lupus Erythematosus: A Systematic Review and Meta-analysis," *Lupus* 23, no. 11 (October 2014): 1156–63.
4. Luis M. Amezcua-Guerra et al., "Joint Involvement in Primary Sjögren's Syndrome: An Ultrasound 'Target Area Approach to Arthritis,'" *Biomed Research International* 2013 (2013): 640265, doi:10.1155/2013/640265.
5. J. W. Smith, P. Chalupa, and M. Shabaz Hasan, "Infectious Arthritis: Clinical Features, Laboratory Findings and Treatment," *Clinical Microbiology and Infection* 12, no. 4 (April 2006): 309–14.

Chapter 5: The Gut-Arthritis Connection

1. Allan M. Mowat and William W. Agace, "Regional Specialization Within the Intestinal Immune System," *Nature Reviews: Immunology* 14 (October 2014): 667–85.
2. Alessio Fasano, "Zonulin and Its Regulation of Intestinal Barrier Function: The Biological Door to Inflammation, Autoimmunity, and Cancer," *Physiological Reviews* 91, no. 1 (January 1, 2011): 151–75.
3. Alessio Fasano, "Leaky Gut and Autoimmune Diseases," *Clinical Reviews in Allergy & Immunology* 42, no. 1 (February 2012): 71–78.
4. Aaron Lerner and Torsten Matthias, "Changes in Intestinal Tight Junction Permeability Associated with Industrial Food Additives Explain the Rising Incidence of Autoimmune Disease," *Autoimmunity Reviews* 14, no. 6 (June 2015): 479–89.
5. Stephen C. Bischoff et al., "Intestinal Permeability: A New Target for Disease Prevention and Therapy," *BMC Gastroenterology* 14 (November 18, 2014): 189.
6. Ibid.
7. Madhukumar Venkatesh et al., "Symbiotic Bacterial Metabolites Regulate Gastrointestinal Barrier Function via the Xenobiotic Sensor PXR and Toll-Like Receptor," *Immunity* 41, no. 2 (August 21, 2014): 296–310.
8. A. Andoh, "Physiological Role of Gut Microbiota for Maintaining Human Health," *Digestion* 93, no. 3 (June 2016): 176–81.

Notes

9. Ron Sender, Shai Fuchs, and Ron Milo, "Are We Really Vastly Outnumbered? Revisiting the Ratio of Bacterial to Host Cells in Humans," *Cell* 164, no. 3 (January 28, 2016): 337–40.

10. Laurence Macia et al., "Microbial Influences on Epithelial Integrity and Immune Function as a Basis for Inflammatory Diseases," *Immunological Reviews* 245, no. 1 (January 2012): 164–76.

11. Ibid.

12. Andrew B. Shreiner, John Y. Kao, and V. Young, "The Gut Microbiome in Health and in Disease," *Current Opinion in Gastroenterology* 31, no. 1 (January 2015): 69–75.

13. Hagit Shapiro et al., "The Cross Talk Between Microbiota and the Immune System: Metabolites Take Center Stage," *Current Opinion in Immunology* 30 (October 2014): 54–62.

14. Andoh, "Physiological Role of Gut Microbiota."

15. Nicholas Arpaia et al., "Metabolites Produced by Commensal Bacteria Promote Peripheral Regulatory T-cell Generation," *Nature* 504, no. 7480 (December 19, 2013): 451–55.

16. Andoh, "Physiological Role of Gut Microbiota"; Alberto Bravo-Blas, Hannah Wessel, and Simon Milling, "Microbiota and Arthritis: Correlations or Cause?," *Current Opinion in Rheumatology* 28, no. 2 (March 2016): 161–67.

17. Shreiner, Kao, and Young, "Gut Microbiome in Health and Disease."

18. Shapiro et al., "Cross Talk Between Microbiota and Immune System."

19. Keiichiro Suzuki and Akira Nakajima, "New Aspects of IgA Synthesis in the Gut," *International Immunology* 26, no. 9 (September 2014): 489–94.

20. N. Bouladoux et al., "Regulatory Role of Suppressive Motifs from Commensal DNA," *Mucosal Immunology* 5, no. 6 (November 2012): 623–34.

21. J. Thorens et al., "Bacterial Overgrowth During Treatment with Omeprazole Compared with Cimetidine: A Prospective Randomised Double Blind Study," *Gut* 39, no. 1 (July 1996): 54–59; Pulukool Sandhya et al., "Does the Buck Stop with the Bugs? An Overview of Microbial Dysbiosis in Rheumatoid Arthritis," *International Journal of Rheumatic Diseases* 19, no. 1 (January 2016): 8–20; Bischoff et al, "Intestinal Permeability."

22. Sandhya et al., "Does the Buck Stop with the Bugs?"

23. R. Shinebaum et al., "Comparison of Faecal Florae in Patients with Rheumatoid Arthritis and Controls," *British Journal of Rheumatology* 26, no. 5 (October 1987): 329–33.

24. Cock et al., "Potential of Selected Australian Medicinal Plants."

25. Yuichi Maeda et al., "Dysbiosis Contributes to Arthritis Development Via Activation of Autoreactive T-cells in the Intestine," *Arthritis & Rheumatology* 68, no. 11 (November 2016): 2646–61.

26. Xuan Zhang et al., "The Oral and Gut Microbiomes Are Perturbed in Rheumatoid Arthritis and Partly Normalized After Treatment," *Nature Medicine* 21, no. 8 (August 2015): 895–905.

27. Sandhya et al., "Does the Buck Stop with the Bugs?"

28. Tejpal Gill et al., "The Intestinal Microbiome in Spondyloarthritis," *Current Opinion in Rheumatology* 27, no. 4 (July 2015): 319–25.

29. Ibid.

30. Jung Min Bae et al., "Association of Inflammatory Bowel Disease with AS and Rheumatoid Arthritis: A Nationwide Population-Based Study," *Modern Rheumatology*, July 26, 2016, doi:10.1080/14397595.2016.1211229.
31. Collins et al., "Relationship Between Inflammation, Gut Microbiota, and Metabolic Osteoarthritis Development."
32. Ursula Fearon et al., "Hypoxia, Mitochondrial Dysfunction and Synovial Invasiveness in Rheumatoid Arthritis," *Nature Reviews: Rheumatology* 12, no. 7 (July 2016): 385–97.
33. Scher et al., "Periodontal Disease and Oral Microbiota"; Bingham and Moni, "Periodontal Disease and Rheumatoid Arthritis."
34. Ketil Moen et al., "Synovial Inflammation in Active Rheumatoid Arthritis and Psoriatic Arthritis Facilitates Trapping of a Variety of Oral Bacterial DNAs," *Clinical and Experimental Rheumatology* 24, no. 6 (November/December 2006): 656–63.

Chapter 6: How to Heal the Gut

1. M. Y. Zeng, N. Inohara, and G. Nuñez, "Mechanism of Inflammation-Driven Bacterial Dysbiosis in the Gut," *Mucosal Immunology* 10 (January 2017): 18–26.
2. Alyssa M. Parian et al., "Nutraceutical Supplements for Inflammatory Bowel Disease," *Nutrition in Clinical Practice* 30, no. 4 (August 2015): 551–58.
3. Elnaz Vaghef-Mehrabany et al., "Probiotic Supplementation Improves Inflammatory Status in Patients with Rheumatoid Arthritis," *Nutrition* 30, no. 4 (April 2014): 430–35.
4. Bedaiwi and Inman, "Microbiome and Probiotics."
5. Beitullah Alipour et al., "Effects of Lactobacillus Casei Supplementation on Disease Activity and Inflammatory Cytokines in Rheumatoid Arthritis Patients: A Randomized Double-Blind Clinical Trial," *International Journal of Rheumatic Diseases* 17, no. 5 (June 2014): 519–27.
6. Maria de los Angeles Pineda et al., "A Randomized, Double-Blinded, Placebo-Controlled Pilot Study of Probiotics in Active Rheumatoid Arthritis," *Medical Science Monitor* 17, no. 6 (June 2011): 347–54.
7. Ehud Baharav et al., "Lactobacillus GG Bacteria Ameliorate Arthritis in Lewis Rats," *Journal of Nutrition* 134, no. 8 (August 2004): 1964–69.
8. Sarika Amdekar et al., "Lactobacillus Acidophilus Protected Organs in Experimental Arthritis by Regulating the Pro-inflammatory Cytokines," *Indian Journal of Clinical Biochemistry* 29, no. 4 (October/December 2014): 471–78.
9. Ibid.
10. Jae-Seon So et al., "Lactobacillus Casei Enhances Type II Collagen/Glucosamine-Mediated Suppression of Inflammatory Responses in Experimental Osteoarthritis," *Life Sciences* 88, nos. 7/8 (February 14, 2011): 358–66.
11. John O'Callaghan et al., "Influence of Adhesion and Bacteriocin Production by *Lactobacillus salivarius* on the Intestinal Epithelial Cell Transcriptional Response," *Applied and Environmental Microbiology* 78, no. 15 (August 2012): 5196–203.
12. Bischoff et al., "Intestinal Permeability."

13. Jean Robert Rapin and Nicolas Wiernsperger, "Possible Links Between Intestinal Permeability and Food Processing: A Potential Therapeutic Niche for Glutamine," *Clinics* 65, no. 6 (June 2010): 635–43.

14. Xiangbing Mao et. al., "Dietary *Lactobacillus rhamnosus* GG Supplementation Improves the Mucosal Barrier Function in the Intestine of Weaned Piglets Challenged by Porcine Rotavirus," *PLoS ONE* 11, no. 1 (January 4, 2016): e0146312. doi:10.1371/journal.pone.0146312.

15. Duan Liu et al., "Effects of Probiotics on Intestinal Mucosa Barrier in Patients with Colorectal Cancer After Operation: Meta-analysis of Randomized Controlled Trials," *Medicine* 95, no. 15 (April 2016): e3342.

16. Colleen R. Kelly et al., "Update on Fecal Microbiota Transplantation 2015: Indications, Methodologies, Mechanisms, and Outlook," *Gastroenterology* 149, no. 1 (July 2015): 223–37; E. G. Pamer, "Fecal Microbiota Transplantation: Effectiveness, Complexities, and Lingering Concerns," *Mucosal Immunology* 7, no. 2 (March 2014): 210–14.

17. Francesca Romana Ponziani, Viviana Gerardi, and Antonio Gasbarrini, "Diagnosis and Treatment of Small Intestinal Bacterial Overgrowth," *Expert Review of Gastroenterology & Hepatology* 10, no. 2 (2016): 215–27.

18. Victor Chedid et al., "Herbal Therapy Is Equivalent to Rifaximin for the Treatment of Small Intestinal Bacterial Overgrowth," *Global Advances in Health and Medicine* 3, no. 3 (May 2014): 16–24.

19. Ibid.

20. Anil Kumar et al., "Current Knowledge and Pharmacological Profile of Berberine: An Update," *European Journal of Pharmacology* 761 (August 15, 2015): 288–97.

21. Yifeng Jin, Daulat B. Khadka, and Won-Jea Cho, "Pharmacological Effects of Berberine and Its Derivatives: A Patent Update," *Expert Opinion on Therapeutic Patents* 26, no. 2 (2016): 229–43.

22. Junling Han, Huiling Lin, and Weiping Huang, "Modulating Gut Microbiota as an Anti-diabetic Mechanism of Berberine," *Medical Science Monitor* 17, no. 7 (July 2011): RA164–67.

23. Yi Cao et al., "Modulation of Gut Microbiota with Berberine Improves Steatohepatitis in High-Fat Diet Fed BALB/C Mice," *Archives of Iranian Medicine* 19, no. 3 (March 2016): 197–203.

24. Kumar et al., "Current Knowledge and Pharmacological Profile of Berberine."

25. F. L. Hu, "Comparison of Acid and Helicobacter pylori in Ulcerogenesis of Duodenal Ulcer Disease," *Zhonghua Yi Xue Za Zhi* 73, no. 4 (April 1993): 217–19, 253.

26. Natural Medicines Professional Datebase, https://naturalmedicines.therapeutic research.com/databases/food,-herbs-supplements/professional.aspx?product id=1126.

27. O. Brorson and S. H. Brorson, "Grapefruit Seed Extract Is a Powerful *In Vitro* Agent Against Motile and Cystic Forms of *Borrelia burgdorferi sensu lato*," *Infection* 35, no. 3 (June 2007): 206–8.

28. Zdenka Cvetnič and Sanda Vladimir-Knezevič, "Antimicrobial Activity of Grapefruit Seed and Pulp Ethanolic Extract," *Acta Pharmaceutica* 54, no. 3 (September 2004): 243–50.

29. G. Ionescu et al., "Oral Citrus Seed Extract in Atopic Eczema: *In Vitro* and *In Vivo* Studies on Intestinal Microflora," *Journal of Orthomolecular Medicine* 5, no. 3 (1990): 155–57.

30. John P. Heggers et al., "The Effectiveness of Processed Grapefruit-Seed Extract as an Antibacterial Agent: II. Mechanism of Action and *In Vitro* Toxicity," *Journal of Alternative and Complementary Medicine* 8, no. 3 (June 2002): 333–40.

31. Anna A. Tolmacheva, Eugene A. Rogozhin, and Dmitry G. Deryabin, "Antibacterial and Quorum Sensing Regulatory Activities of Some Traditional Eastern-European Medicinal Plants," *Acta Pharmaceutica* 64, no. 2 (June 2014): 173–86.

32. Natural Medicines Professional Database, https://naturalmedicines.therapeu ticresearch.com/databases/food,-herbs-supplements/professional.aspx?prod uctid=350.

33. Sayed H. Abidi et al., "Synergy Between Antibiotics and Natural Agents Results in Increased Antimicrobial Activity Against *Staphylococcus epidermidis*," *Journal of Infection in Developing Countries* 9, no. 9 (September 27, 2015): 925–29.

34. Ryszard Amarowicz, Gary A. Dykes, and Ronald B. Pegg, "Antibacterial Activity of Tannin Constituents from *Phaseolus vulgaris, Fagoypyrum esculentum, Corylus avellana* and *Juglans nigra*," *Fitoterapia* 79, no. 3 (April 2008): 217–19.

35. Natural Medicines Professional Database, https://naturalmedicines.therapeutic research.com/databases/food,-herbs-supplements/professional.aspx?product id=639.

36. Monika Derda et al., "*Artemisia annua* L. as a Plant with Potential Use in the Treatment of Acanthamoebiasis," *Parasitology Research* 115 (2016): 1635–39.

37. Fabien Juteau et al., "Antibacterial and Antioxidant Activities of *Artemisia annua* Essential Oil," *Fitoterapia* 73, no. 6 (October 2002): 532–35.

38. Liwang Cui and Xin-zhuan Su, "Discovery, Mechanisms of Action and Combination Therapy of Artemisinin," *Expert Review of Anti-infective Therapy* 7, no. 8 (October 2009): 999–1013.

39. Elisa Bona et al., "Sensitivity of *Candida albicans* to Essential Oils: Are They an Alternative to Antifungal Agents?," *Journal of Applied Microbiology* 121, no. 6 (December 2016): 1530–45.

40. Aghil Sharifzadeh and Hojjatollah Shokri, "Antifungal Activity of Essential Oils from Iranian Plants Against Fluconazole-Resistant and Fluconazole-Susceptible *Candida albicans*," *Avicenna Journal of Phytomedicine* 6, no. 62 (March/April 2016): 215–22.

41. I. H. Soares et al., "In Vitro Activity of Essential Oils Extracted from Condiments Against Fluconazole-Resistant and -Sensitive *Candida glabrata*," *Journal of Medical Mycology* 25, no. 3 (September 2015): 213–17.

42. Mark Force, William S. Sparks, and Robert A. Ronzio, "Inhibition of Enteric Parasites by Emulsified Oil of Oregano *In Vivo*," *Phytotherapy Research* 14, no. 3 (May 2000): 213–14.

43. Rapin and Wiernsperger, "Possible Links Between Intestinal Permeability and Food Processing."

44. Julien Bertrand et al., "Glutamine Restores Tight Junction Protein Claudin-1 Expression in Colonic Mucosa of Patients with Diarrhea-Predominant Irri-

table Bowel Syndrome," *Journal of Parenteral and Enteral Nutrition* 40, no. 8 (November 2016): 1170–76.

45. Xiaoliang Shu et al., "Glutamine Decreases Intestinal Mucosal Injury in a Rat Model of Intestinal Ischemia-Reperfusion by Downregulating HB1 and Inflammatory Cytokine Expression," *Experimental and Therapeutic Medicine* 12, no. 3 (September 2016): 1367–72.

46. Ibtissem Ghouzali et al., "Targeting Immunoproteasome and Glutamine Supplementation Prevent Intestinal Hyperpermeability," *Biochimica et Biophysica Acta* 1861, no. 1, pt. A (January 2017): 3278–88.

47. Geraldo E. Vicentini et al., "Experimental Cancer Cachexia Changes Neuron Numbers and Peptide Levels in the Intestine: Partial Protective Effects After Dietary Supplementation with L-Glutamine," *PloS One* 11, no. 9 (September 16, 2016): e0162998.

48. Natural Medicines Professional Database, https://naturalmedicines.therapeutic research.com/databases/food,-herbs-supplements/professional.aspx?product id=878.

49. Parian et al., "Nutraceutical Supplements for Inflammatory Bowel Disease."

50. Rapin and Wiernsperger, "Possible Links Between Intestinal Permeability and Food Processing."

51. Shuying Tian et al., "Curcumin Protects Against the Intestinal Ischemia-Reperfusion Injury: Involvement of the Tight Junction Protein ZO-1 and TNF-α Related Mechanism," *Korean Journal of Physiology & Pharmacology* 20, no. 2 (March 2016): 147–52.

52. Rita-Marie T. McFadden et al., "The Role of Curcumin in Modulating Colonic Microbiota During Colitis and Colon Cancer Prevention," *Inflammatory Bowel Diseases* 21, no. 11 (November 2015): 2483–94.

53. Na Wang et al., "Resveratrol Protects Oxidative Stress-Induced Intestinal Epithelial Barrier Dysfunction by Upregulating Heme Oxygenase-1 Expression," *Digestive Diseases and Sciences* 61, no. 9 (September 2016): 2522–34.

54. Sonja Skrovanek et al., "Zinc and Gastrointestinal Disease," *World Journal of Gastrointestinal Pathophysiology* 5, no. 4 (November 15, 2014): 496–513.

55. Mary Carmen Valenzano et al., "Remodeling of Tight Junctions and Enhancement of Barrier Integrity of the CACO-2 Intestinal Epithelial Cell Layer by Micronutrients," *PLoS One* 10, no. 7 (July 30, 2015): e0133926.

Chapter 7: Food and Fire

1. Loren Cordain et al., "Origins and Evolution of the Western Diet: Health Implications for the 21st Century," *American Journal of Clinical Nutrition* 81, no. 2 (February 2005): 341–54.

2. Ibid.

3. Ibid.

4. Ibid.

5. Ibid.

6. D. L. Katz and S. Meller, "Can We Say What Diet Is Best for Health?," *Annual Review of Public Health* 35 (2014): 83–103.

7. Ibid.
8. María M. Adeva and Gema Souto, "Diet-Induced Metabolic Acidosis," *Clinical Nutrition* 30, no. 4 (August 2011): 416–21.
9. Ramy Abdelhamid and Kathleen Sluka, "ASICs Mediate Pain and Inflammation in Musculoskeletal Diseases," *Physiology* 30, no. 6 (November 2015): 449–59.
10. H. A. Mousa, "Health Effects of Alkaline Diet and Water, Reduction of Digestive-Tract Bacterial Load, and Earthing," *Alternative Therapies in Health and Medicine* 22 (supplement 1) (April 2016): 24–33.
11. Nathalie Poupin et al., "Impact of the Diet on Net Endogenous Acid Production and Acid-Base Balance," *Clinical Nutrition* 31, no. 3 (June 2012): 313–21.
12. Katz and Meller. "Can We Say What Diet Is Best for Health?"
13. J. Gordon Millichap and Michelle M. Yee, "The Diet Factor in Attention-Deficit/Hyperactivity Disorder," *Pediatrics* 129, no. 2 (February 2012): 330–37.
14. Hannah Louise Simpson and Barry J. Campbell, "Dietary Fibre–Microbiota Interactions," *Alimentary Pharmacology and Therapeutics* 42, no. 2 (July 2015): 158–79.
15. Juana I. Mosele, Alba Macià, and Maria-José Motilva, "Metabolic and Microbial Modulation of the Large Intestine Ecosystem by Non-Absorbed Diet Phenolic Compounds: A Review," *Molecules* 20, no. 9 (September 18, 2015): 17429–68;
16. Simpson and Campbell, "Dietary Fibre–Microbiota Interactions."
17. Marcel Roberfroid et al., "Prebiotic Effects: Metabolic and Health Benefits," *British Journal of Nutrition* 104 (supplement 2) (August 2010): S1–S63.
18. Kenji Shinohara et al., "Effect of Apple Intake on Fecal Microbiota and Metabolites in Humans," *Anaerobe* 16, no. 5 (October 2010): 510–15.
19. Jiacheng Huang et al., "Different Flavonoids Can Shape Unique Gut Microbiota Profile In Vitro," *Journal of Food Science* 81, no. 9 (September 2016): H2273–79.
20. Tugba Ozdal et al., "The Reciprocal Interactions Between Polyphenols and Gut Microbiota and Effects on Bioaccessibility," *Nutrients* 8, no. 2 (February 2016): 78.
21. Marta Wlodarska et al., "Phytonutrient Diet Supplementation Promotes Beneficial Clostridia Species and Intestinal Mucus Secretion Resulting in Protection Against Enteric Infection," *Scientific Reports* 5 (last modified March 19, 2015), doi:2932/10.1038/srep09253.
22. Zeng, Inohara, and Nuñez, "Mechanism of Inflammation-Driven Bacterial Dysbiosis."
23. Andoh, "Physiological Role of Gut Microbiota"; Bravo-Blas, Wessel, and Milling, "Microbiota and Arthritis."
24. Johanna Maukonen and Maria Saarela, "Human Gut Microbiota: Does Diet Matter?," *Proceedings of the Nutrition Society* 74, no. 1 (February 2015): 23–36.
25. Melanie Uhde et al., "Intestinal Cell Damage and Systemic Immune Activation in Individuals Reporting Sensitivity to Wheat in the Absence of Coeliac Disease," *Gut*, published online July 25, 2016, doi:10.1136/gutjnl-2016-311964.
26. Lisa K. Stamp, Michael J. James, and Leslie G. Cleland, "Diet and Rheumatoid

Arthritis: A Review of the Literature," *Seminars in Arthritis and Rheumatism* 35, no. 2 (October 2005): 77–94.

27. Geir Smedslund et al., "Effectiveness and Safety of Dietary Interventions for Rheumatoid Arthritis: A Systematic Review of Randomized Controlled Trials," *Journal of the American Dietetic Association* 110, no. 5 (May 2010): 727–35.

28. Stamp, James, and Cleland, "Diet and Rheumatoid Arthritis"; R. Peltonen et al., "Changes of Faecal Flora in Rheumatoid Arthritis During Fasting and One-Year Vegetarian Diet," *British Journal of Rheumatology* 33, no. 7 (July 1994): 638–43.

29. Bravo-Blas, Wessel, and Milling, "Microbiota and Arthritis."

30. R. Peltonen et al., "Faecal Microbial Flora and Disease Activity in Rheumatoid Arthritis During a Vegan Diet," *British Journal of Rheumatology* 36, no. 1 (January 1997): 64–68.

31. J. Kjeldsen-Kragh, "Rheumatoid Arthritis Treated with Vegetarian Diets," *American Journal of Clinical Nutrition* 70, no. 3 (supplement 3) (September 1999): 594S–600S.

32. Stamp, James, and Cleland, "Diet and Rheumatoid Arthritis."

33. Clinton et al., "Whole-Foods, Plant-Based Diet."

34. David J. Hunter et al., "The Intensive Diet and Exercise for Arthritis (IDEA) Trial: 18-Month Radiographic and MRI Outcomes," *Osteoarthritis and Cartilage* 23, no. 7 (July 2015): 1090–98.

Chapter 8: Traumatic Stress: Fueling the Flame

1. Shanta R. Dube et al., "Cumulative Childhood Stress and Autoimmune Diseases in Adults," *Psychosomatic Medicine* 71, no. 2 (February 2009): 243–50.

2. Joseph A. Boscarino, Christopher W. Forsberg, and Jack Goldberg, "A Twin Study of the Association Between PTSD Symptoms and Rheumatoid Arthritis," *Psychosomatic Medicine* 72, no. 5 (June 2010): 481–86.

3. Ibid.

4. Aoife O'Donovan et al., "Current Posttraumatic Stress Disorder and Exaggerated Threat Sensitivity Associated with Elevated Inflammation in the Mind Your Heart Study," *Brain, Behavior, and Immunity* 60 (February 2017): 198–205.

Chapter 10: 3-Step Arthritis Protocol and Guide

1. Hector L. Lopez, "Nutritional Interventions to Prevent and Treat Osteoarthritis, Part 1: Focus on Fatty Acids and Macronutrients," *PM&R* 4 (supplement 5) (May 2012): S145–S154.

2. B. Galarraga et al., "Cod Liver Oil (*n*-3 Fatty Acids) as an Non-steroidal Anti-inflammatory Drug Sparing Agent in Rheumatoid Arthritis," *Rheumatology* 47, no. 5 (May 2008): 665–69.

3. Melainie Cameron, Joel J. Gagnier, and Sigrun Chrubasik, "Herbal Therapy for Treating Rheumatoid Arthritis," Cochrane Database of Systematic Reviews (February 16, 2011): CD002948. doi:10.1002/14651858.CD002948.pub2.

Notes

4. Dragan Vasiljevic et al., "Valuation of the Effects of Different Supplementation on Oxidative Status in Patients with Rheumatoid Arthritis," *Clinical Rheumatology* 35, no. 8 (August 2016): 1909–15.

5. Yunes Panahi, "Mitigation of Systemic Oxidative Stress by Curcuminoids in Osteoarthritis: Results of a Randomized Controlled Trial," *Journal of Dietary Supplements* 13, no. 2 (2015): 209–20.

6. Gilberto Fabián Hurtado-Torres, Lourdes Larisa González-Baranda, and Carlos Abud-Mendoza, "Rheumatoid Cachexia and Other Nutritional Alterations in Rheumatologic Diseases," *Rheumatología Clínica* 11, no. 5 (September/October 2015): 316–21.

7. Quiñonez-Flores, "Oxidative Stress Relevance in the Pathogenesis of the Rheumatoid Arthritis"; Somaiya Mateen et al., "Increased Reactive Oxygen Species Formation and Oxidative Stress in Rheumatoid Arthritis," *PLoS One* 11, no. 4: e0152925. Published: April 4, 2016, http://dx.doi.org/10.1371/journal.pone.0152925.

8. Romina R. Riveiro-Naveira et al., "Resveratrol Lowers Synovial Hyperplasia, Inflammatory Markers and Oxidative Damage in an Acute Antigen-Induced Arthritis Model," *Rheumatology* 55, no. 10 (October 2016): 1889–1900.

9. Hani M. Khojah et al., "Reactive Oxygen and Nitrogen Species in Patients with Rheumatoid Arthritis as Potential Biomarkers for Disease Activity and the Role of Antioxidants," *Free Radical Biology & Medicine* 97 (August 2016): 285–91.

10. Larissa Lumi Watanabe Ishikawa et al., "Vitamin D Deficiency and Rheumatoid Arthritis," *Clinical Reviews in Allergy & Immunology* (2016): doi:10.1007/s12016-016-8577-0.

Index

Index

Index

Index

About the Author

A true pioneer in functional medicine, Susan Blum, M.D., M.P.H., an assistant clinical professor in the Department of Preventive Medicine at the Icahn School of Medicine at Mount Sinai, has been treating, healing, and preventing chronic diseases for nearly two decades. Her passion and dedication for identifying and addressing the root causes of chronic illness through the groundbreaking whole-body approach known as functional medicine has helped thousands of people and is transforming our health care system.

A preventive medicine and chronic disease specialist, Dr. Blum is the founder and director of Blum Center for Health in Rye Brook, New York, where she leads a large, multispecialty team of physicians, nurse practitioners, nutritionists, and health coaches, all providing cutting-edge functional and integrative medicine services. Dr. Blum brings the collective experience and wisdom from both her own medical practice and that of the team to her books and online programs. This strong foundation of expertise explains why her programs are so successful.

In her first bestselling book, *The Immune System Recovery Plan* (Scribner, 2013), Dr. Blum offers her four-step program, which she has used to help thousands of patients recover from autoimmune and immune-related conditions without medication. Dr. Blum also created an online companion for the Immune System Recovery Plan to provide additional support. She recently launched a new digital platform, BlumHealthMD.com, to expand these programs by including a targeted HealMyGut Program and providing individual and group coaching. Dr. Blum's second book, *Healing Arthritis* (Scribner, 2017), offers a unique, groundbreaking approach to helping arthritis sufferers reverse and even heal this condition. As a companion to her new book, Dr. Blum has created a comprehensive online program, the Arthritis Action Plan.

As part of her vision to help people adopt a healthier lifestyle, Dr. Blum cofounded Organic Pharmer, a healthy grab-and-go food and juice café that opened in 2014, where she oversees all menu items to make sure they follow the principles of functional medicine. Today Organic Pharmer has two locations in New York but delivers nationwide.

Dr. Blum is a member of the medical advisory board for *The Dr. Oz Show* and the Institute for Integrative Nutrition and a senior teaching faculty with the Center for Mind-Body Medicine in Washington, DC, and teaches throughout the world in its training programs. She is also on the board of directors for the American College of Lifestyle Medicine's True Health Initiative. She has appeared on *The Dr. Oz Show, Fox 5 News*, and *ABC Eyewitness News*, and is regularly quoted in *Real Simple, Harper's Bazaar*, and *Redbook*, among other publications.

Dr. Blum is on the medical staff at Greenwich Hospital, completed her internal medicine training at St. Luke's–Roosevelt Hospital and her residency in preventive medicine at the Icahn School of Medicine at Mount Sinai in New York City. Board certified in preventive medicine and integrative and holistic medicine, she received her master's in public health at Columbia University and her certification in functional medicine from the Institute for Functional Medicine in Gig Harbor, Washington.

Dr. Blum approaches medicine—and her life—from a whole-body perspective, incorporating all facets of wellness into every aspect. She begins each day with a twenty-minute meditation, a green smoothie made from the contents of her garden, and a walk on her country road with her dog, Trixie. She lives in Armonk, New York, with her husband and has three grown sons.